THE
ULTIMATE
BULLWORKER
REP RANGE
WORKOUTS
BOOK THREE

The ULTIMATE BULLWORKER REP RANGE WORKOUTS

BOOK THREE

The Best Isotonic Exercises to build muscle, increase strength, power and sculpt the best body with the power of Isometrics!

BECOME A BULLWORKER MAN!

The Ultimate Bullworker Rep Range Workouts Book Three was written to help you get closer to your physical potential when it comes to real muscle sculpting strengthening exercises. The exercises and routines in this book are quite demanding, so consult your physician and have a physical exam taken prior to the start of this exercise program. Proceed with the suggested exercises and information at your own risk. The Publishers and author shall not be liable or responsible for any loss, injury, or damage allegedly arising from the information or suggestions in this book.

The Ultimate Bullworker Rep Range Workouts Book Three[1]
a muscle-building master-plan

By

Birch Tree Publishing
Published by Birch Tree Publishing

Birch Tree Publishing

Dedication

To all Bullworker men and women, **GET TRANSFORMED NOW!**

Contents

A Powerful Body Starts Here

Build "Muscles" NOW!

The Bullworker Rep Range Book Three is the fastest muscle-producing program EVER!

Introduction by Marlon Birch CSCS

Trainees of the Bullworker Power Series" know that we present the best muscle-building programs to increase optimum strength and add quality to one's life. That's my ultimate goal with my muscle enhancing programs.

This book introduces The Ultimate Power Rep Range Series these programs will get you in the best shape **FASTER** than you thought possible. With the power of our system and the muscle-building benefits of isometrics holds. Combining Isotonics and Isometrics forces the muscles to contract harder and over come neuromuscular system failure.

Our methods extend a set beyond failure, and you will see muscle popping up almost overnight. While getting more muscular and leaner than ever before. It's an eye-opening program that can help you pack on muscle and strength fast. We also look at the optimal rep speed for you to keep building muscles while applying various factors to increase growth.

Keep moving forward

Marlon Birch
Yours In Health and Strength

FULL-BODY

WORKOUTS

CHAPTER 1

REP RANGE

PHASE ONE

2 WEEKS

REP SPEED CONTRACT 2 SECONDS, RELEASE 2 SECONDS

01 REP RANGE PHASE ONE

Day 1 and 2 perform 30 reps per set
Day 3 and 4 perform 10 reps per set
Day 5 and 6 perform 30 reps per set
Perform all exercises without rest. Alternate day 1 and two for 6 days per week.
Rounds 3 Isometric contraction 30 seconds per exercise on the last rep.

DAY ONE

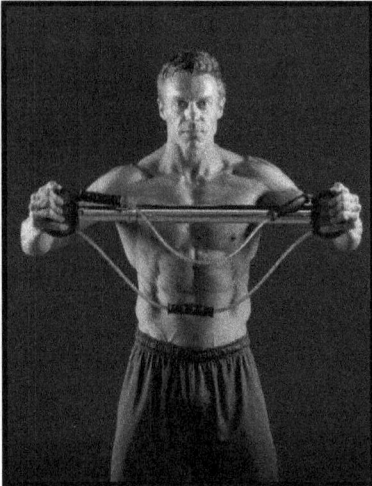
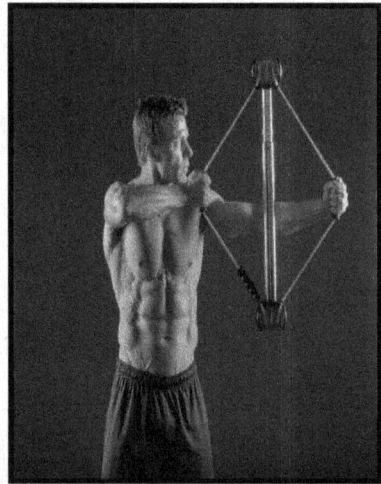

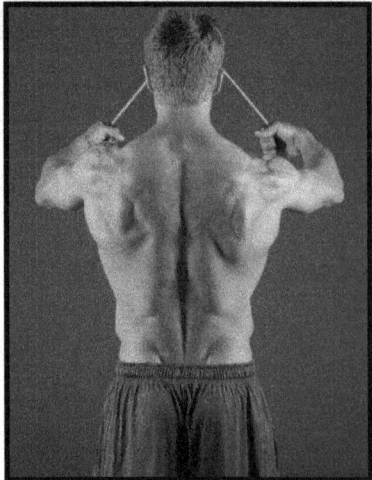
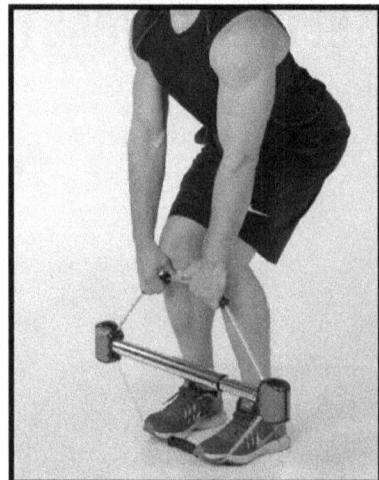

01 REP RANGE PHASE ONE

DAY ONE CONTINUED.....

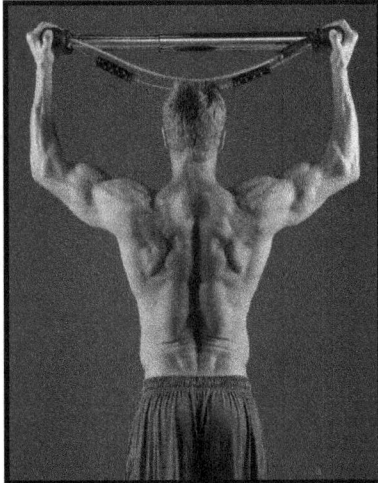

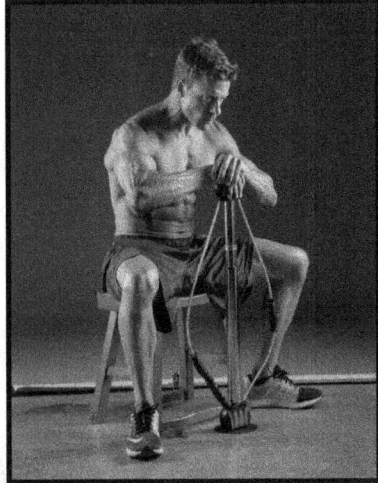

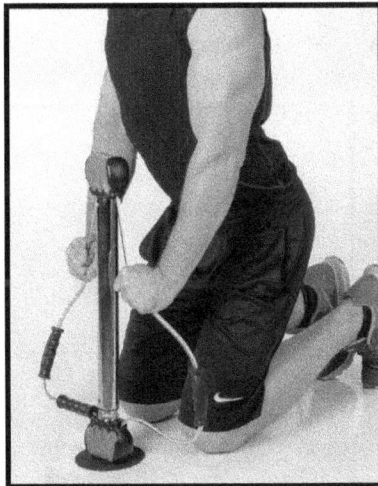

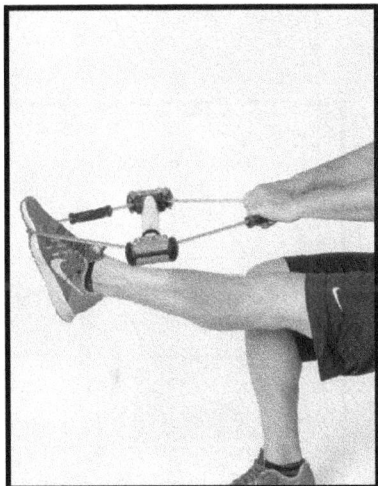

01 REP RANGE PHASE ONE

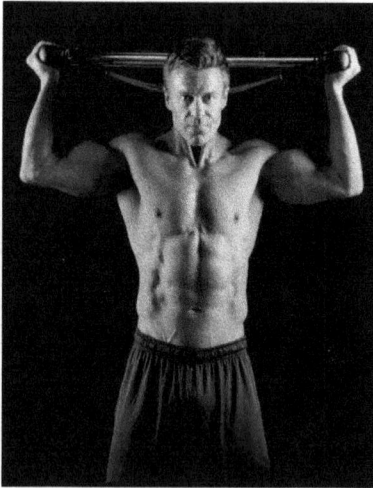

TWO CONTI

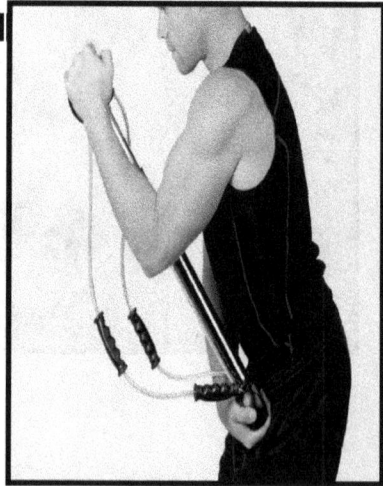

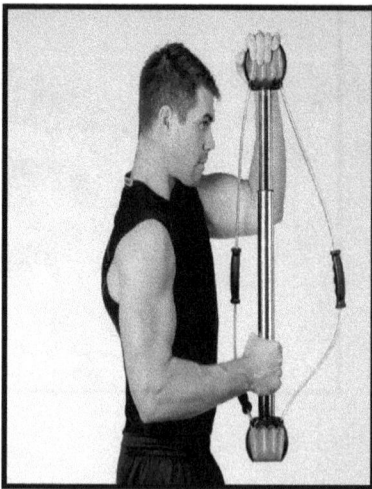

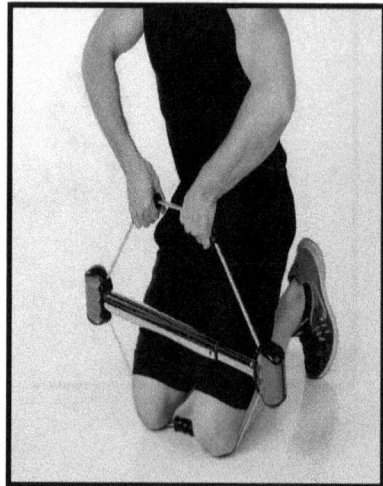

01 STANDARD PROGRAM

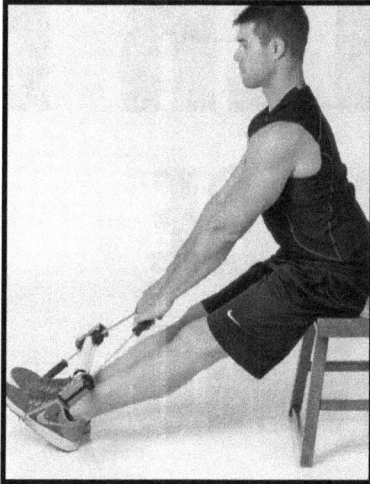

TWO CONT

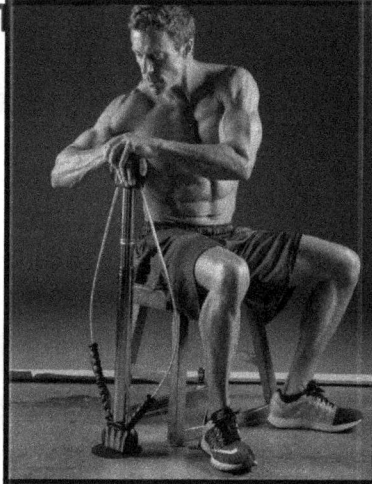

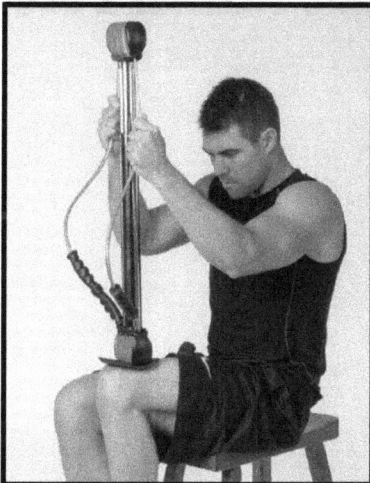

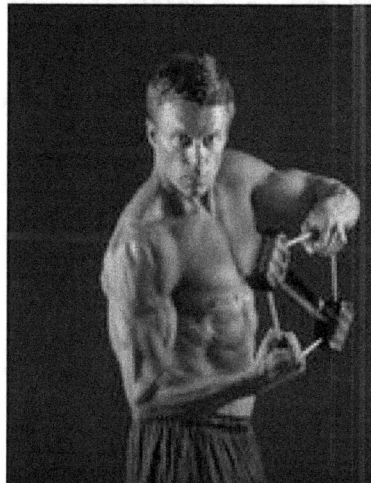

CHAPTER 1
REP RANGE

PHASE TWO

2 WEEKS
REP SPEED CONTRACT 2 SECONDS, RELEASE 2 SECONDS

01 REP RANGE

Day 1 and 2 perform 5-7 reps per set
Day 3 and 4 perform 10 reps per set
Day 5 and 6 perform 20 reps per set
Perform all exercises without rest. Alternate day 1 and two for 6 days per week.
Rounds 3 Isometric contraction 15 seconds per exercise on the last rep.

DAY ONE

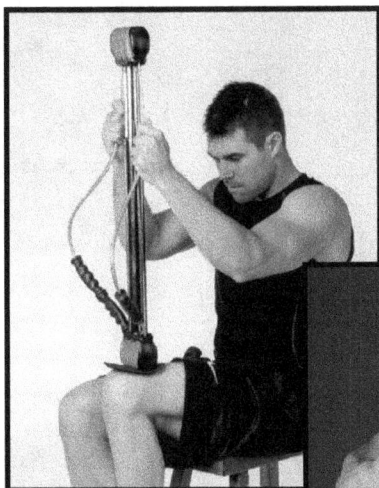
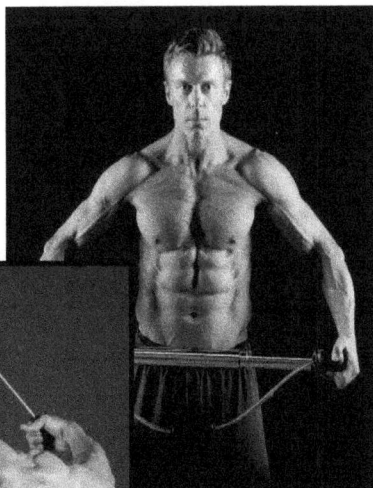
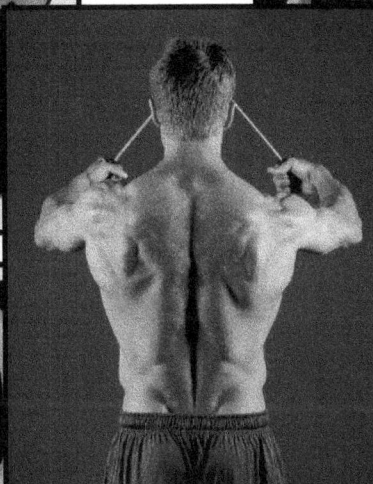
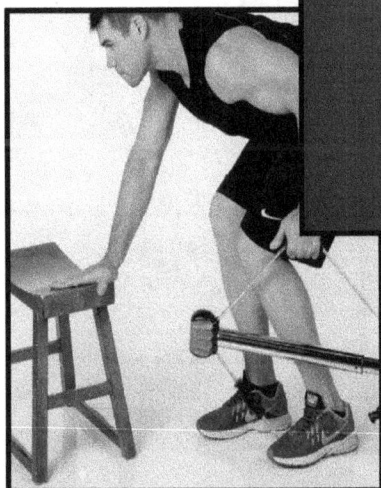
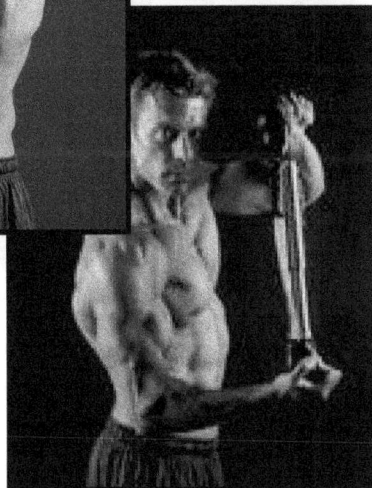

01 STANDARD PROGRAM

DAY TWO

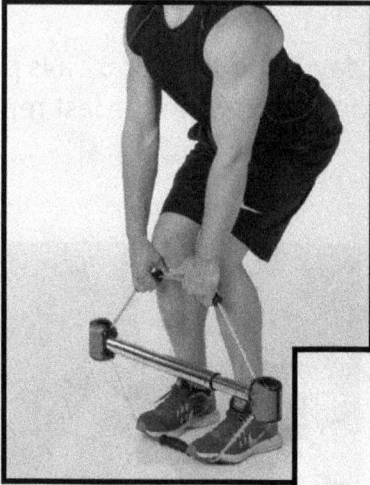
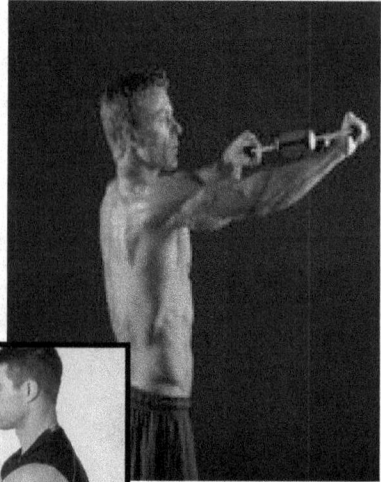
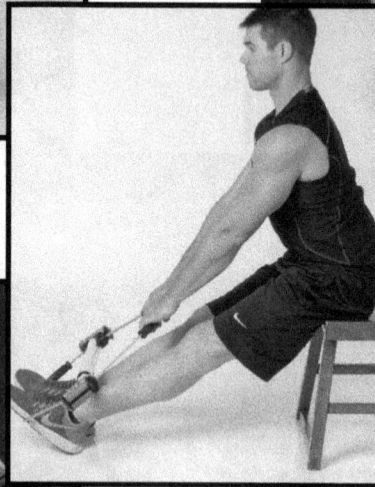
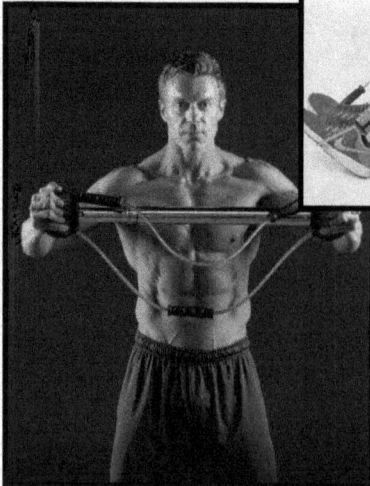
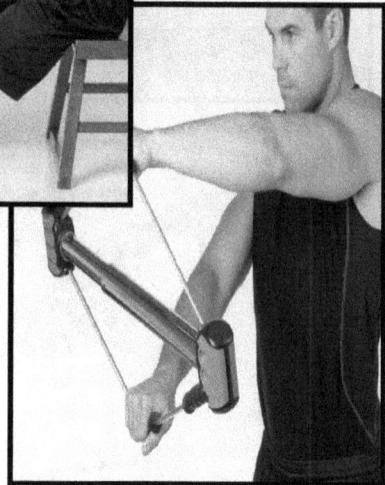

CHAPTER 2
POWER REP RANGE
PHASE THREE
2 WEEKS
REP SPEED CONTRACT 2 SECOND, RELEASE 6 SECONDS

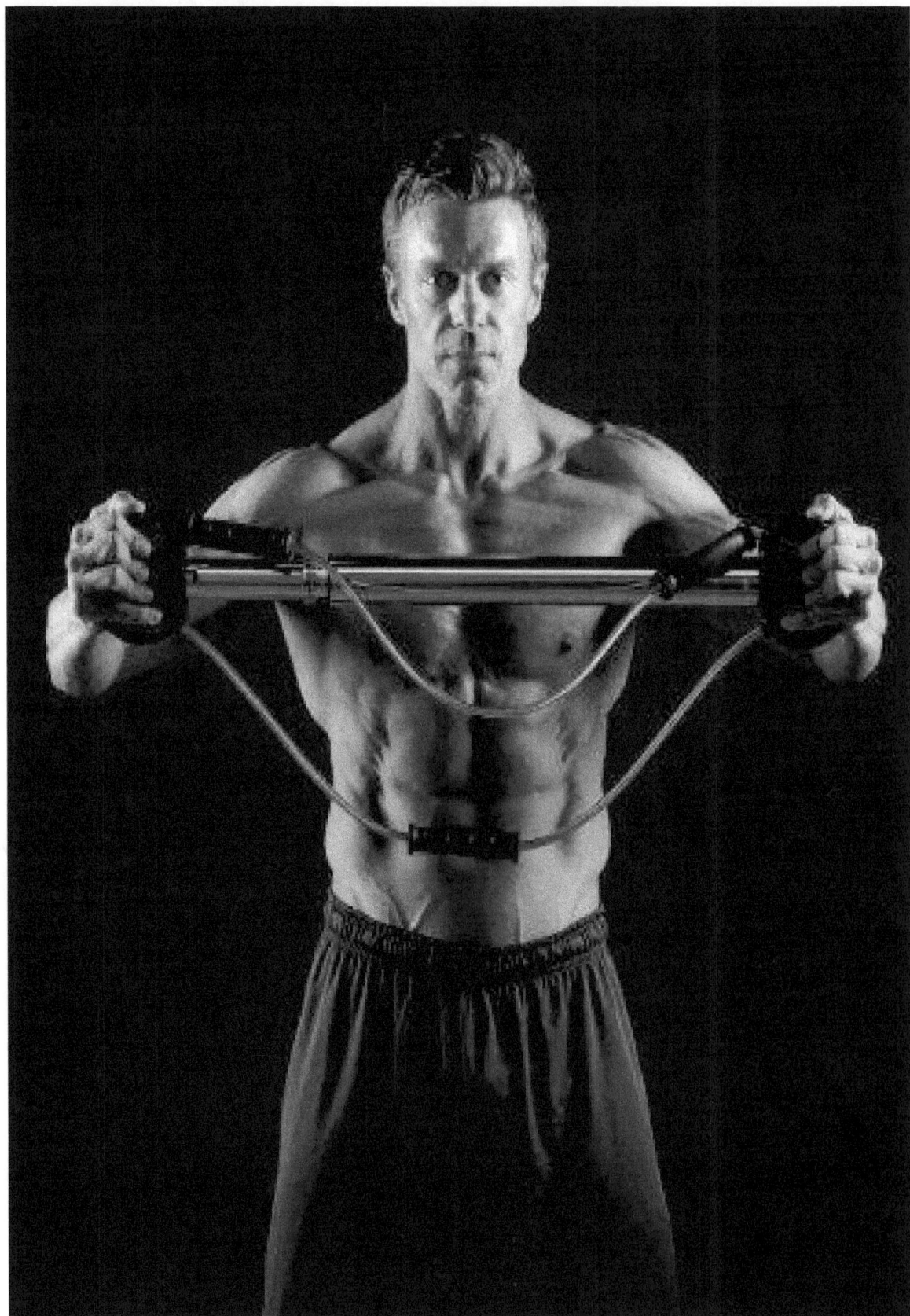

02 POWER REP PROGRAM

All exercises are done non-stop. Perform 7 reps per body part at 4 sets each. followed by a 5 second isometric contraction on each rep.

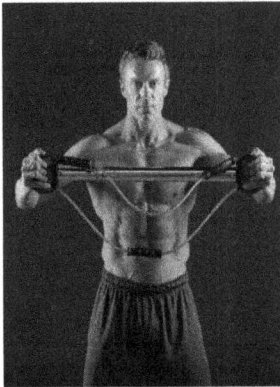
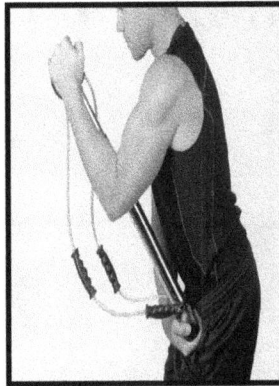
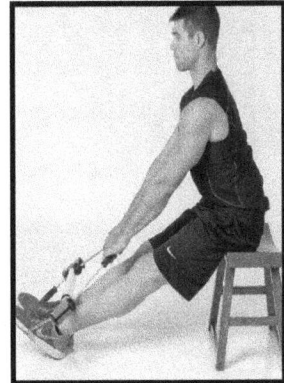

MON, WED, FRI

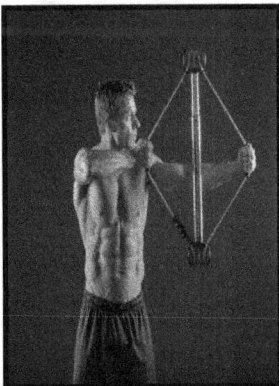
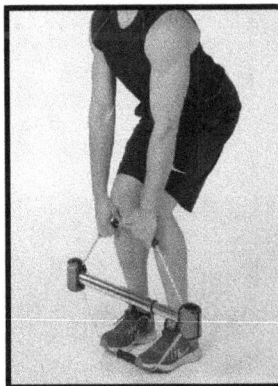
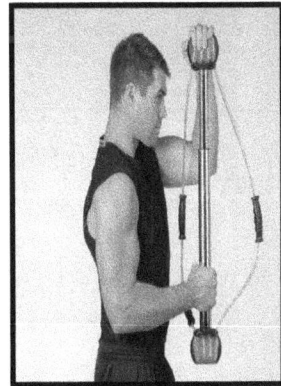

02 POWER REP RANGE PROGRAM

All exercises are done non-stop. Perform 7 reps per body part at 4 sets each. followed by a 5 second isometric contraction on each rep.

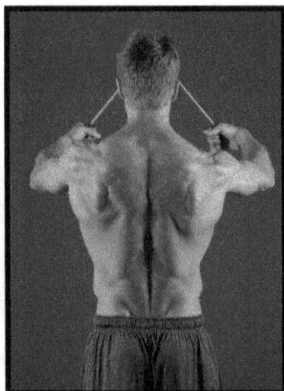

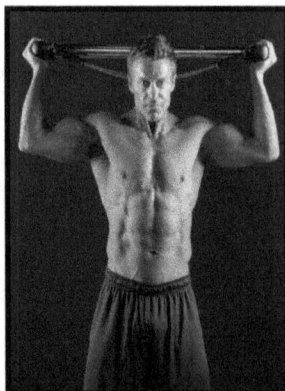

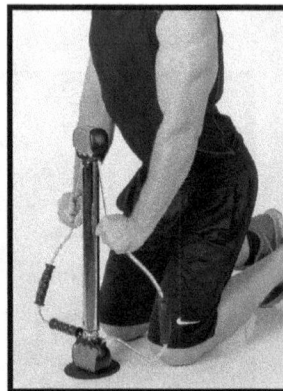

TUES, THURS, SAT

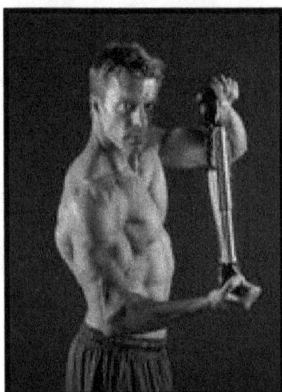

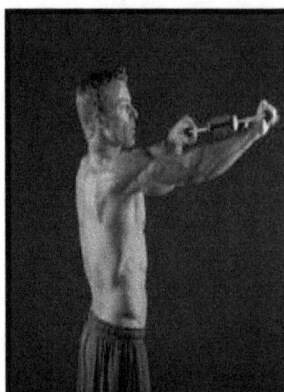

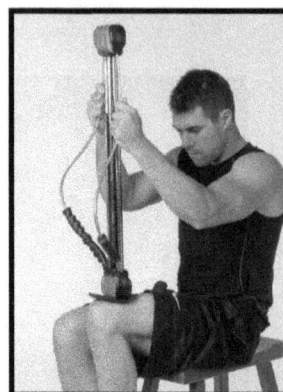

CHAPTER 2
POWER REP RANGE
PHASE FOUR
2 WEEKS
REP SPEED CONTRACT 1 SECOND, RELEASE 2 SECONDS

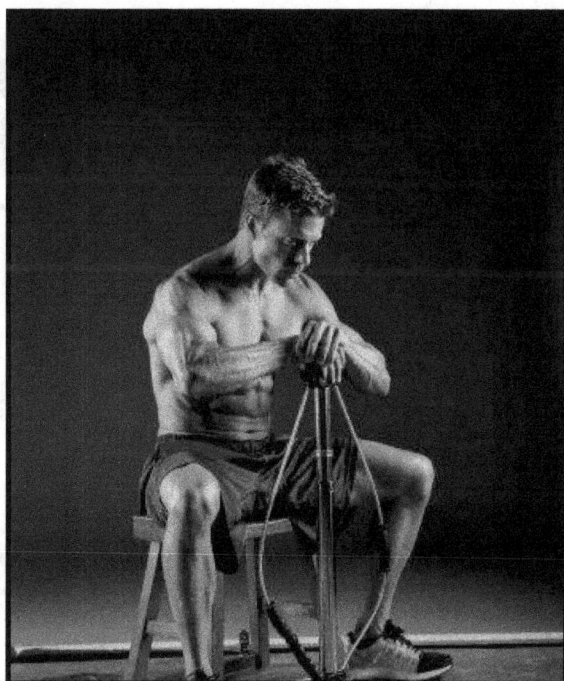

02 POWER REP RANGE PROGRAM

Perform 15 reps, followed by a 30 second isometric contraction. Three sets each exercise. All exercises are done non stop until one round is finished. Rest 5 seconds between rounds.

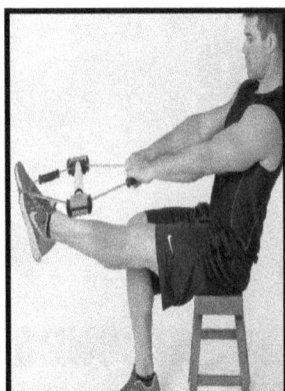
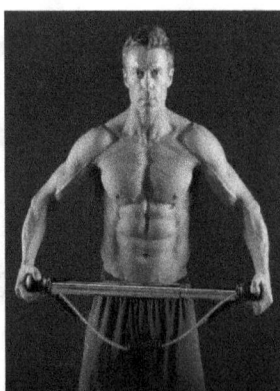
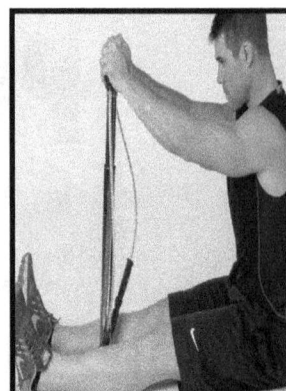

MON, WED, FRI

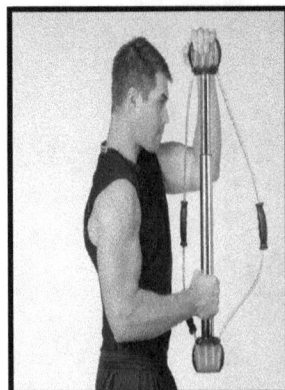
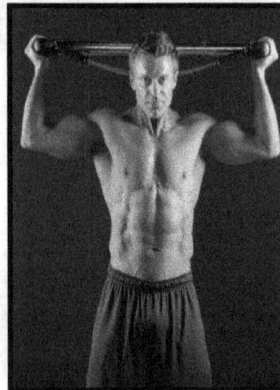
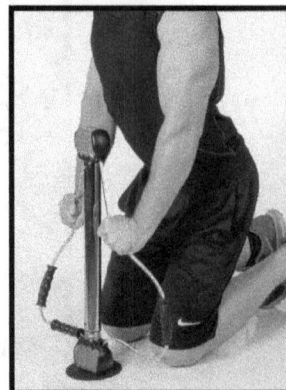

02 POWER REP RANGE PROGRAM

Perform 20 reps, followed by a 20 second isometric contraction. Three sets each exercise. All exercises are done non stop until one round is finished. Rest 5 seconds between rounds.

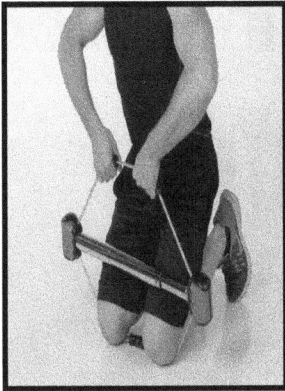

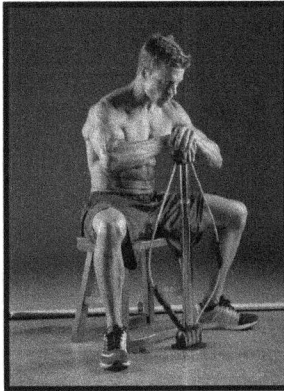

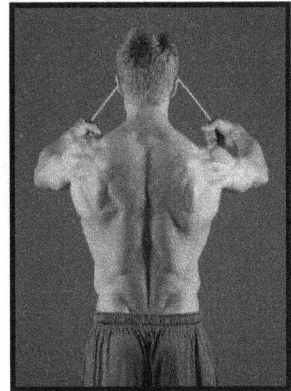

TUES, THURS, SAT

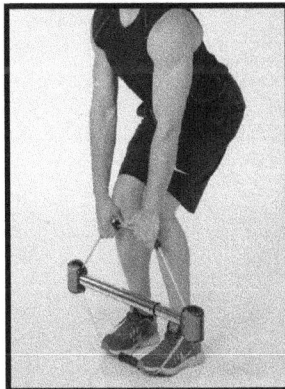

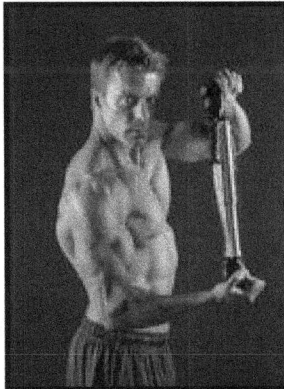

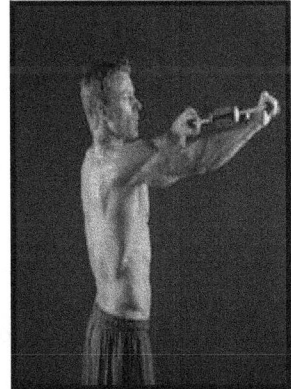

CHAPTER 3
POWER PUMP REP RANGE
PHASE FIVE
2 WEEKS
REP SPEED CONTRACT 2 SECONDS, RELEASE 2 SECONDS

03 POWER PUMP REP RANGE PROGRAM

Perform a 10 second Isometric contraction, followed by 20 reps. On the 20th rep perform an isometric contraction for 30 seconds. Perform all exercises non-stop until one full round is completed. Rest 10 seconds and complete a total of 4 rounds.

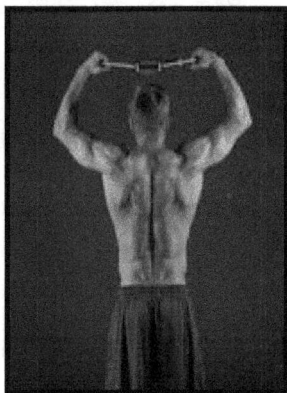
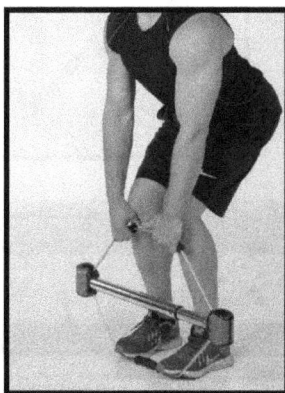
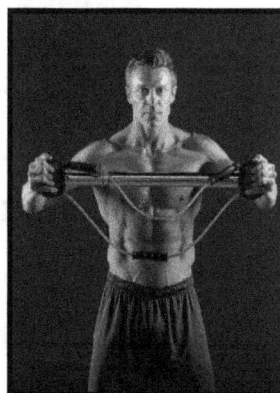

MON, WED, FRI

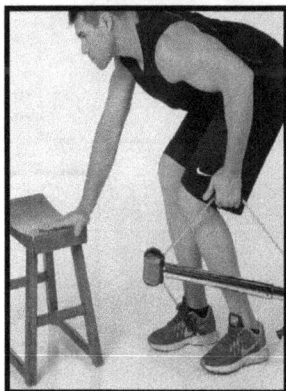
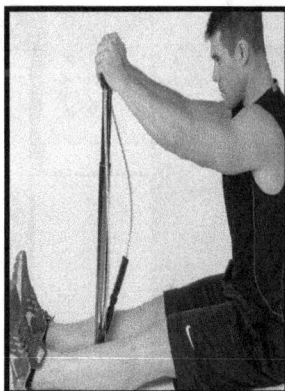
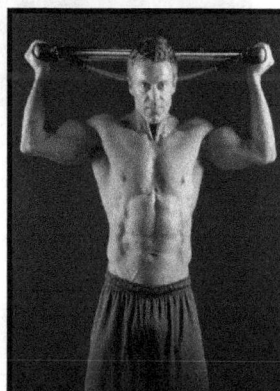

03 POWER PUMP REP RANGE PROGRAM

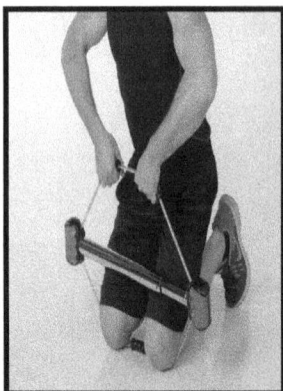

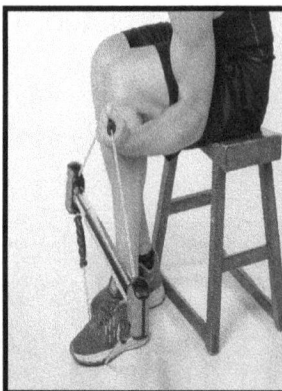

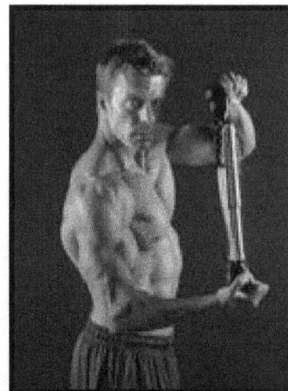

TUES, THURS, SAT

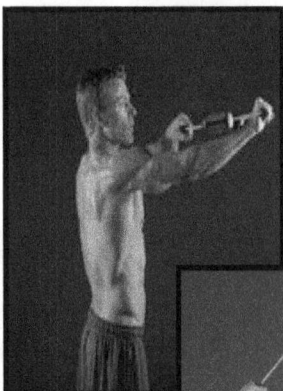

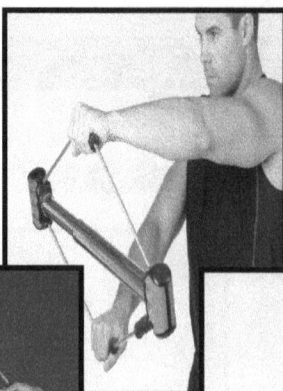

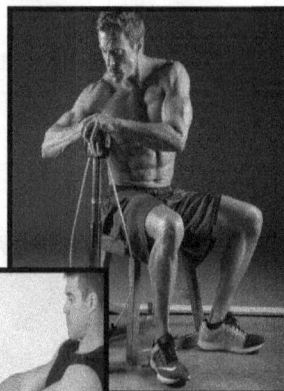

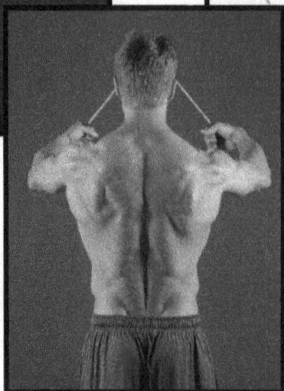

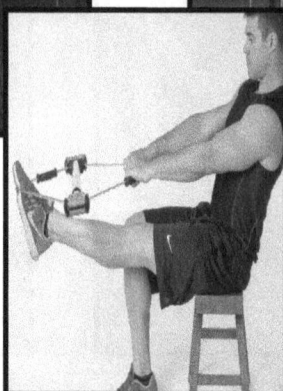

CHAPTER 3
POWER PUMP REP RANGE
PHASE SIX
2 WEEKS
REP SPEED CONTRACT 1 SECOND, RELEASE 3 SECONDS

03 POWER PUMP REP RANGE PROGRAM

Perform a 20 second Isometric contraction, followed by 9 reps. On the 9th rep perform a 25 second isometric contraction. Perform all exercises non-stop until one full round is completed. Rest 10 seconds and complete 4 rounds.

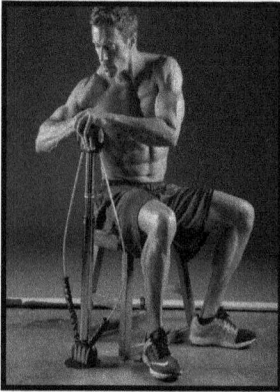 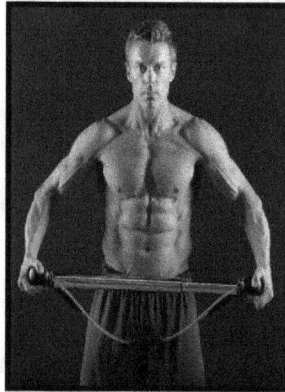 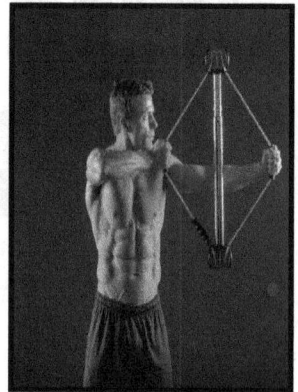

MON, WED, FRI

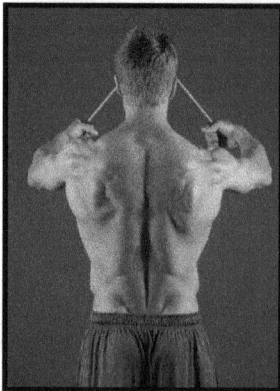 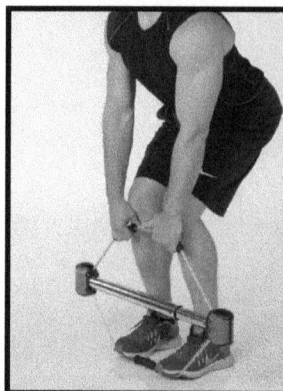 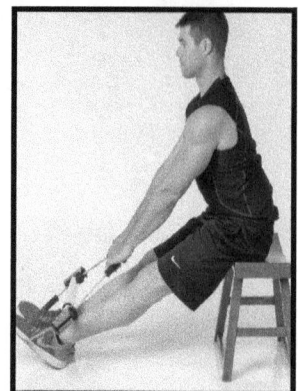

03 POWER PUMP REP RANGE PROGRAM

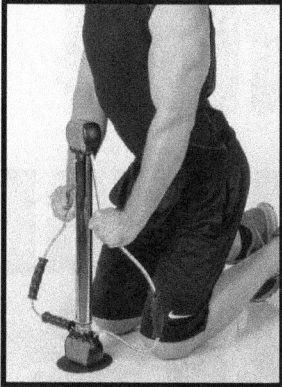

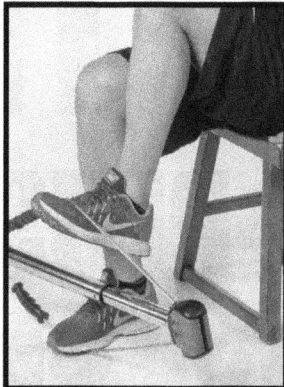

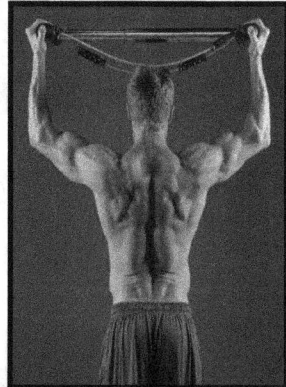

TUES, THURS, SAT

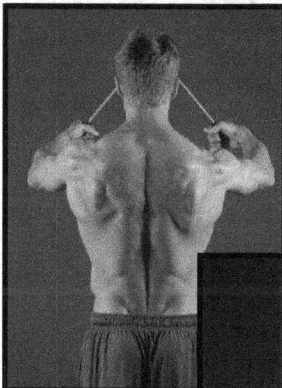

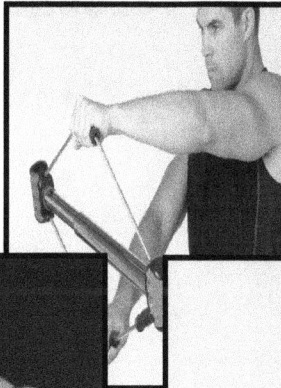

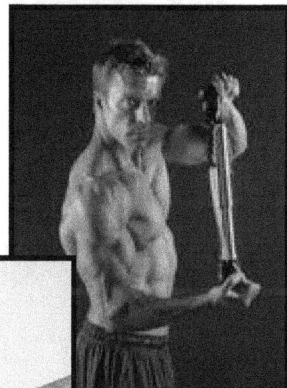

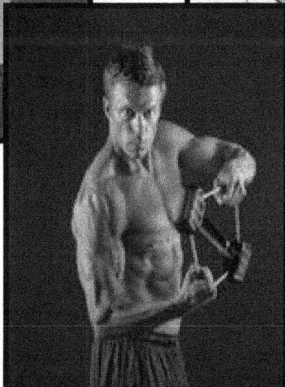

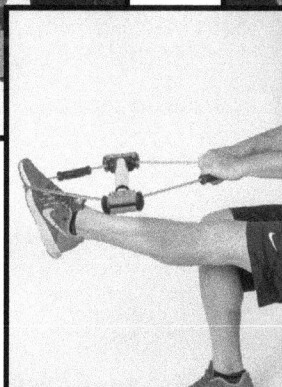

CHAPTER 4
POWER PLUS RANGE
PHASE SEVEN
3 WEEKS
REP SPEED CONTRACT 1 SECOND, RELEASE 6 SECONDS

04 POWER PLUS RANGE PROGRAM

Perform 10 reps. On the 10th rep perform a 15 second isometric contraction continue until all body parts are completed. Perform 2-3 rounds.

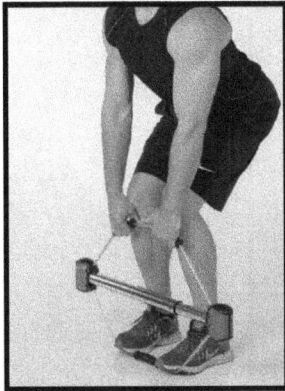 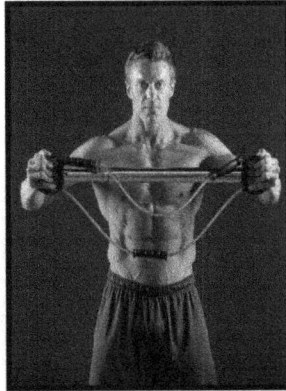 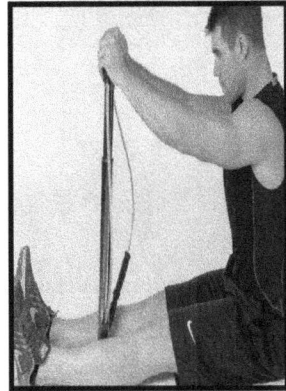

MON, WED, FRI

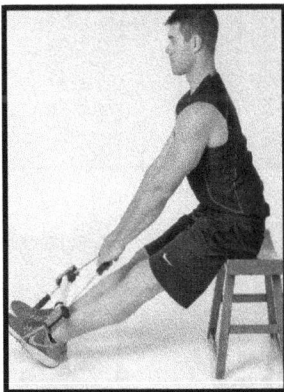 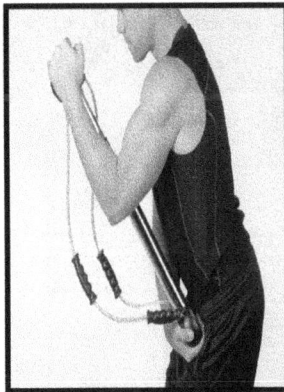 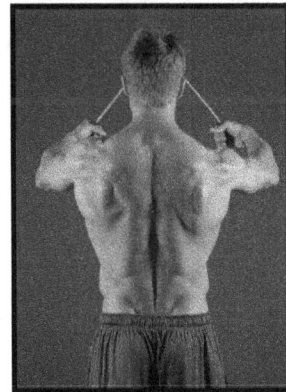

04 POWER PLUS RANGE PROGRAM

On each exercise perform 10 reps. At the end of each rep range perform a 10 second isometric contraction. Continue until all body parts are completed. Perform 3-4 rounds.

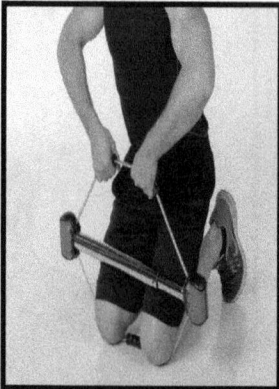

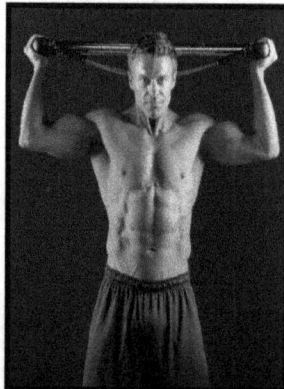

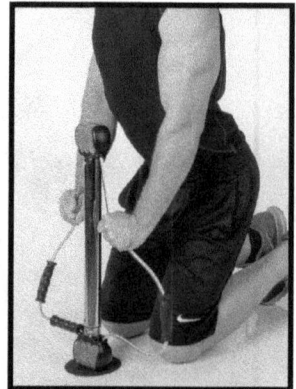

TUES, THURS, SAT

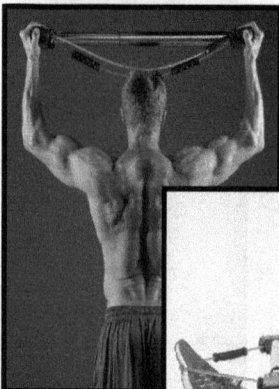

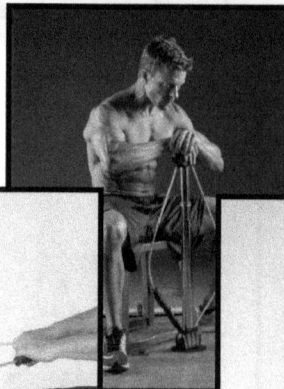

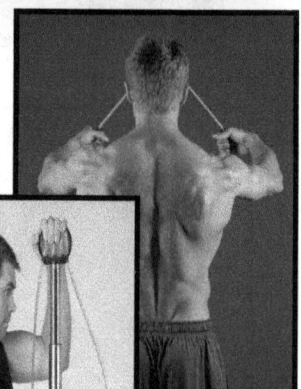

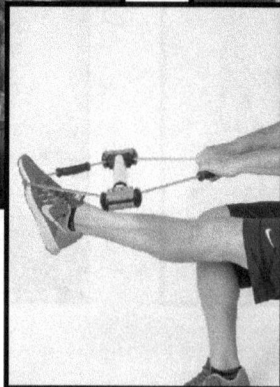

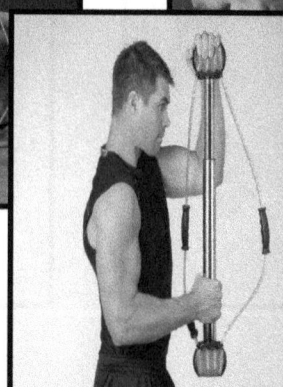

CHAPTER 5
POWER REP
POWER & STRENGTH
PHASE EIGHT
2 WEEKS

REP SPEED CONTRACT 1 SECOND, RELEASE 2 SECONDS
REP RANGES CHANGES WITHIN THE WEEK.

POWER AND STRENGTH PROGRAM

05 POWER AND STRENGTH PROGRAM DAY ONE

HOW TO PERFORM THIS ROUTINE: Perform a 7 second isometric contraction followed by 20 reps per exercise. Perform all exercises non-stop.
PERFORM THREE ROUNDS (SETS)

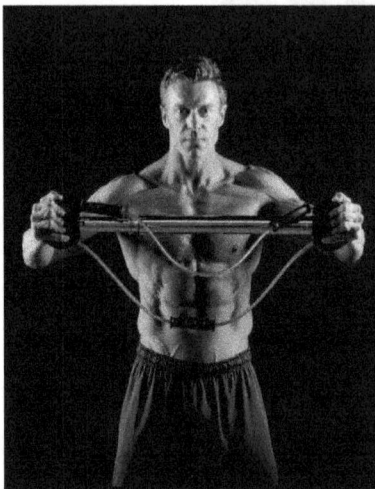

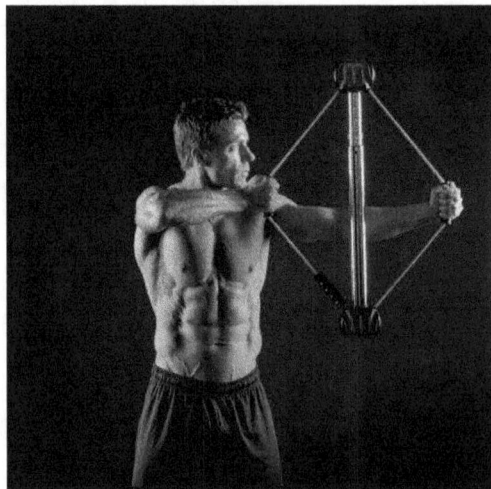

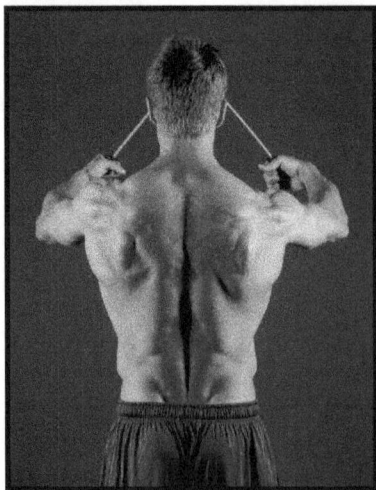

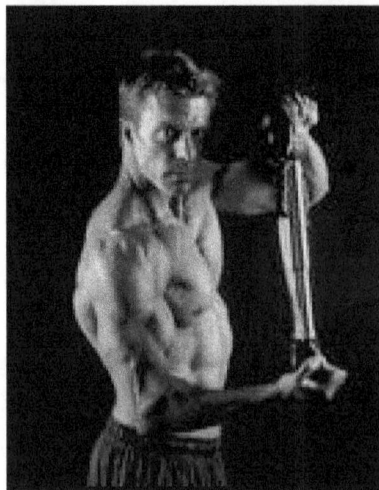

POWER AND STRENGTH PROGRAM

05 POWER AND STRENGTH PROGRAM DAY TWO

HOW TO PERFORM THIS ROUTINE: Perform a 20 second isometric contraction followed by 5-9 reps per exercise. Perform all exercises non-stop.
PERFORM THREE ROUNDS (SETS)

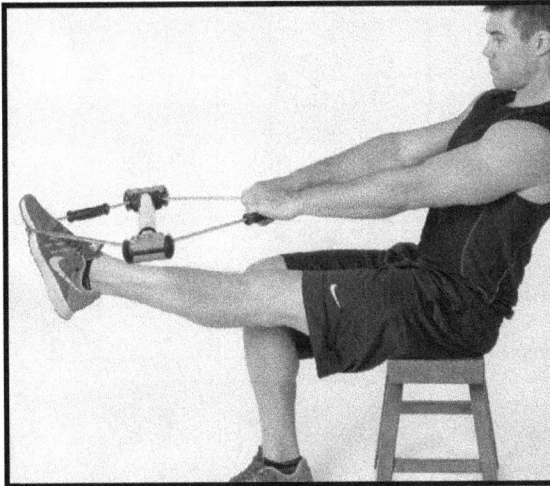

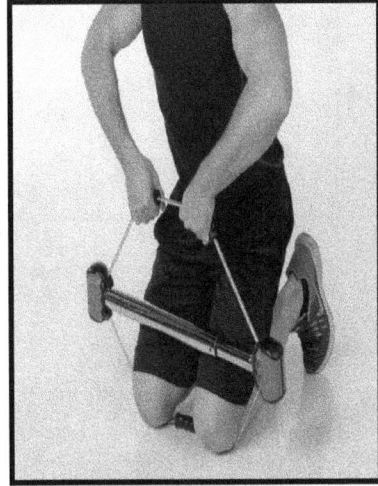

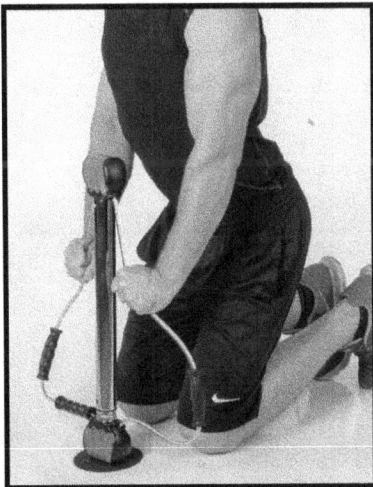

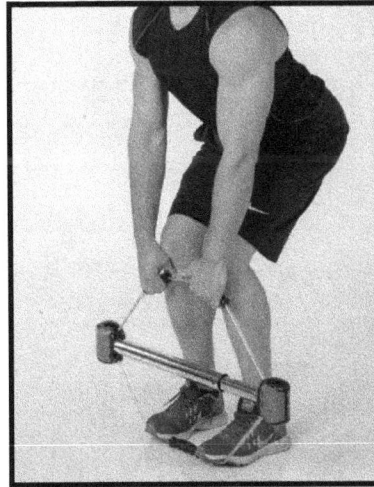

POWER AND STRENGTH PROGRAM

05 POWER AND STRENGTH PROGRAM DAY THREE

HOW TO PERFORM THIS ROUTINE: Perform a 7 second isometric contraction followed by 10 reps per exercise. Perform all exercises non-stop.
PERFORM THREE ROUNDS (SETS)

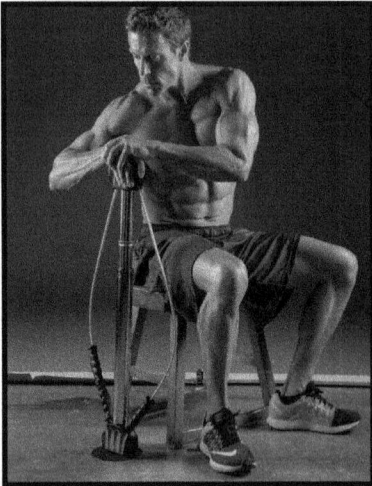

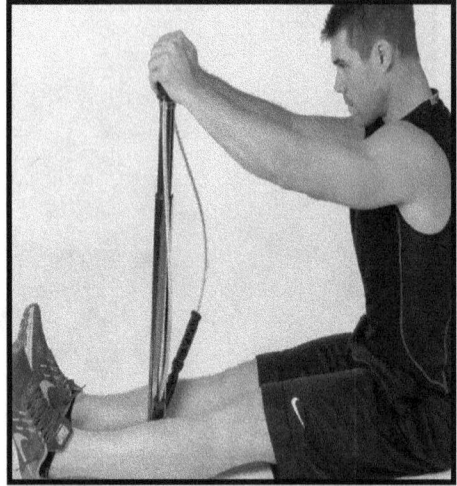

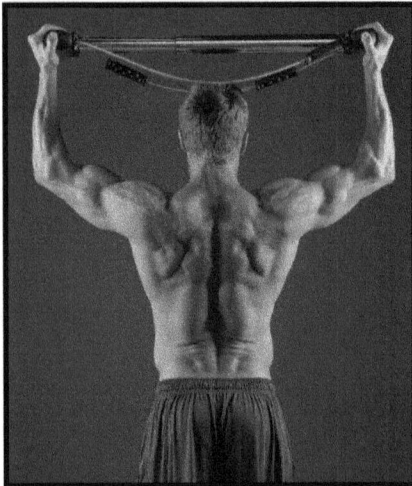

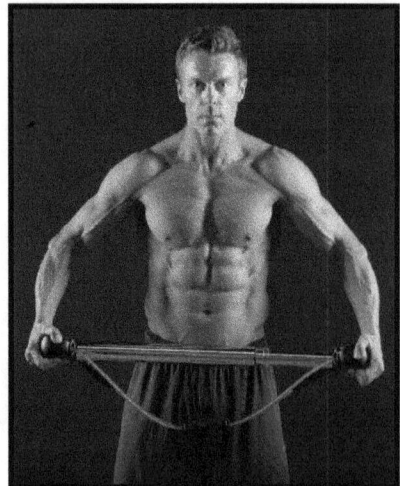

POWER AND STRENGTH PROGRAM

05 POWER AND STRENGTH PROGRAM DAY FOUR

HOW TO PERFORM THIS ROUTINE: Perform a 20 second isometric contraction followed by 30 reps per exercise. Perform all exercises non-stop.
PERFORM THREE ROUNDS (SETS)

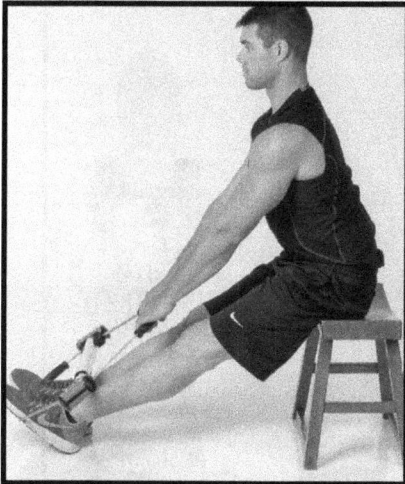

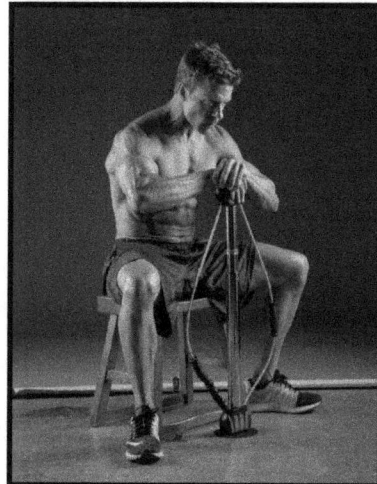

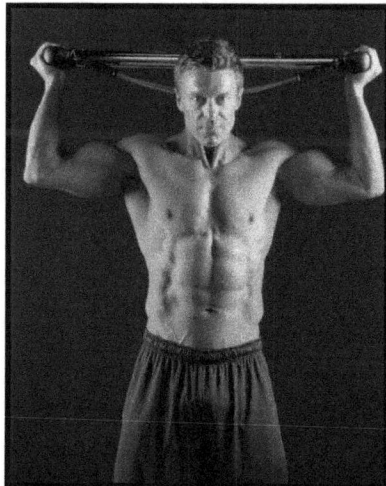

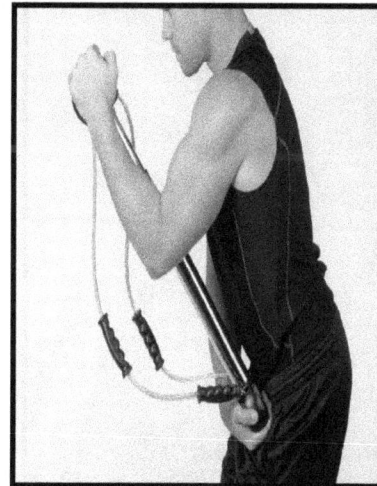

POWER AND STRENGTH PROGRAM

05 POWER AND STRENGTH PROGRAM DAY FIVE

HOW TO PERFORM THIS ROUTINE: Perform a 30 second isometric contraction followed by 20 reps per exercise. Perform all exercises non-stop.
PERFORM THREE ROUNDS (SETS)

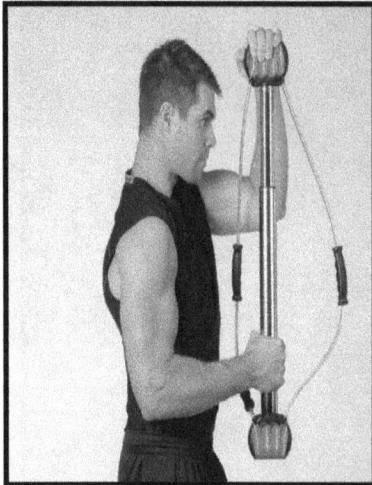

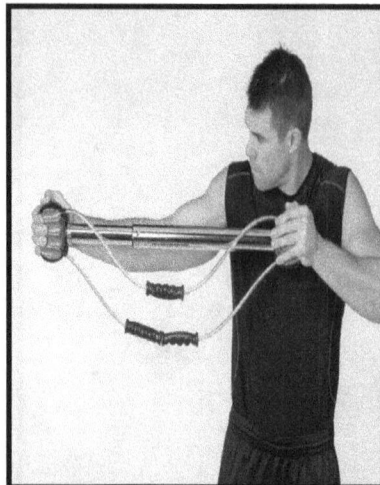

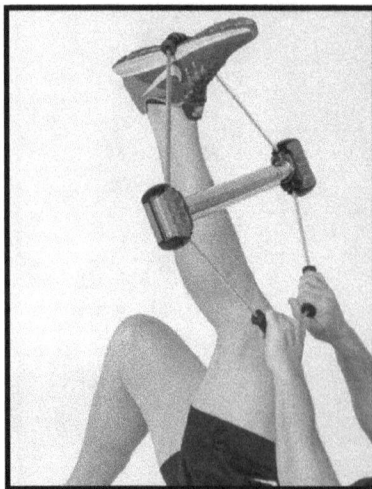

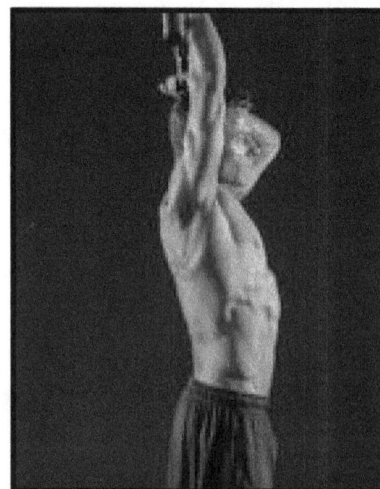

POWER PLUS PROGRAM

06 POWER PLUS STRENGTH PROGRAM

MONDAY, WEDNESDAY, FRIDAY
HOW TO PERFORM THIS ROUTINE: You contract for 1 second and release 2 seconds. Perform 7-9 reps; each rep perform an isometric contraction for 10 seconds. Perform 4 rounds.
Perform plan for 2 weeks before moving to Phase Ten.

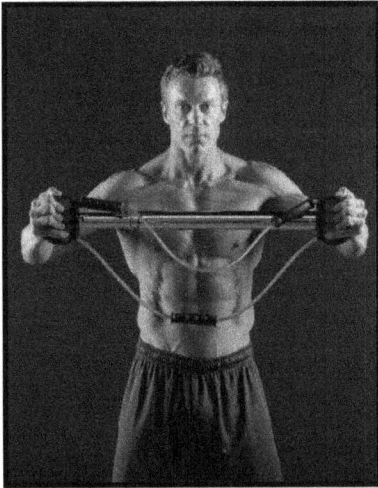
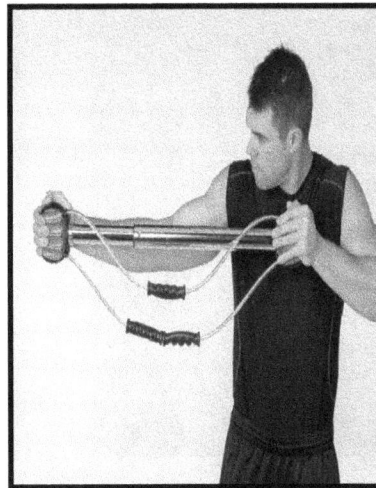
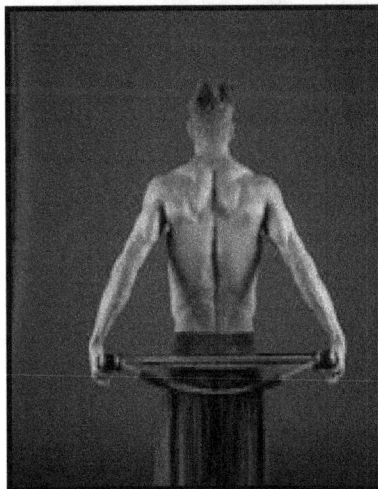
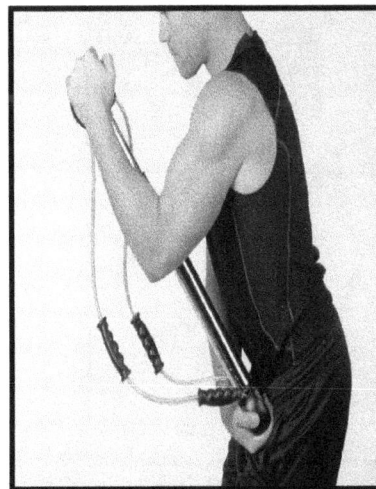

POWER PLUS PROGRAM

06 POWER PLUS STRENGTH PROGRAM

MONDAY,WEDNESDAY,FRIDAY
Routine continued............

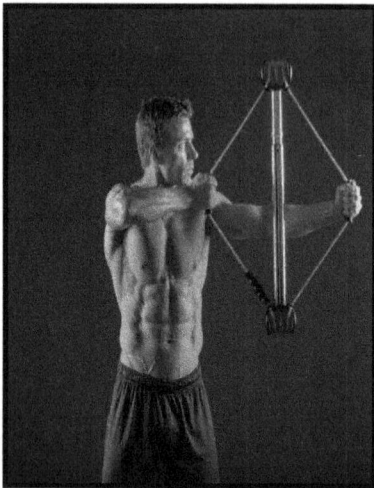

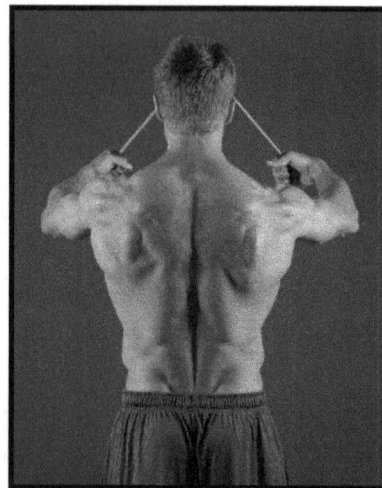

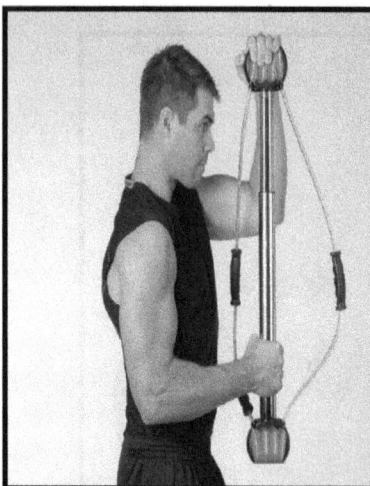

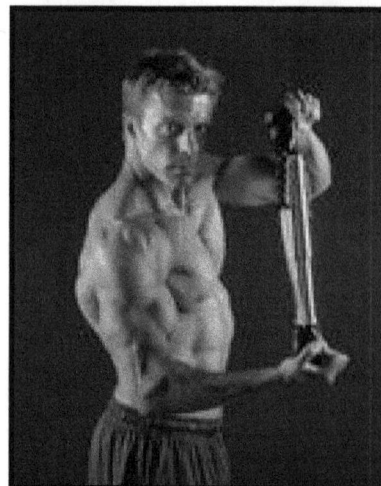

POWER PLUS PROGRAM

06 POWER PLUS STRENGTH PROGRAM

MONDAY, WEDNESDAY, FRIDAY
Routine continued.............

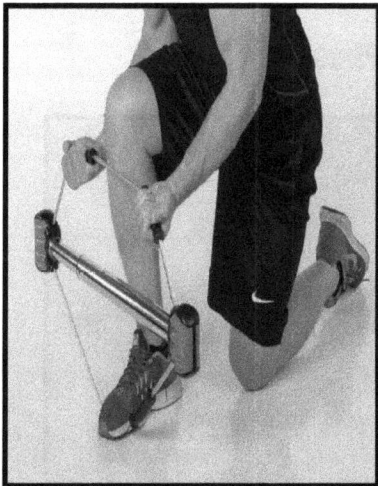

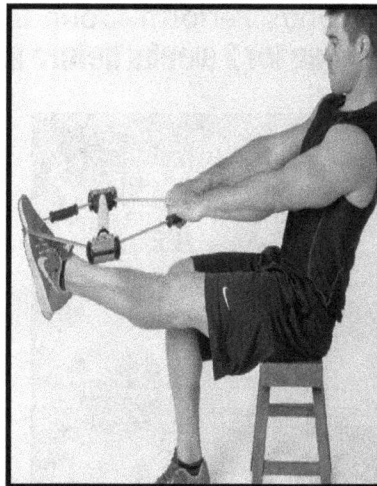

PHASE NINE MON, WED, FRI

POWER PLUS PROGRAM

06 POWER PLUS STRENGTH PROGRAM

TUESDAY, THURSDAY, SATURDAY
HOW TO PERFORM THIS ROUTINE: You contract for 2 seconds and release for a slow 6 seconds. Perform 5-7 reps; each rep perform an isometric contraction for 10 seconds. Perform 4 rounds.
Perform plan for 2 weeks before moving to Phase Ten.

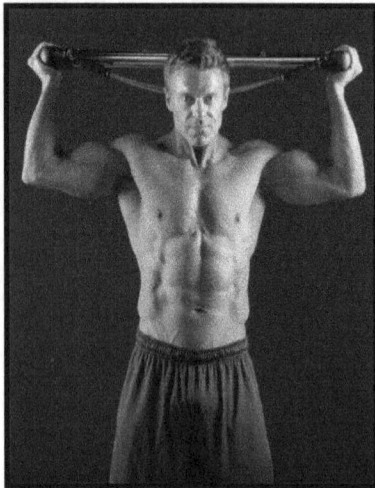

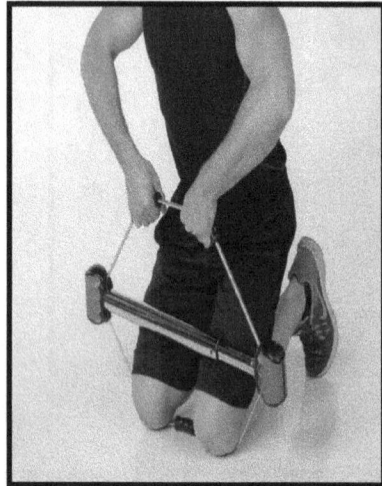

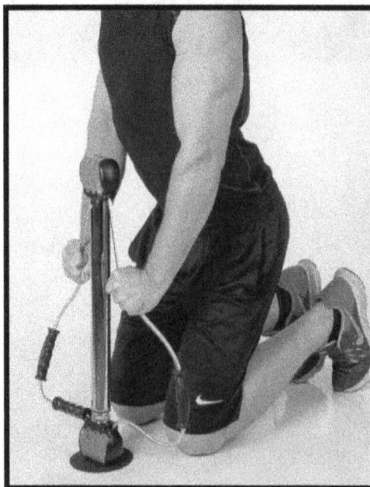

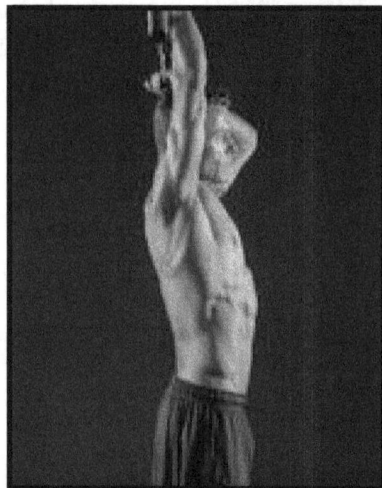

POWER PLUS PROGRAM

06 POWER PLUS STRENGTH PROGRAM

TUESDAY, THURSDAY, SATURDAY
Routine continued...................

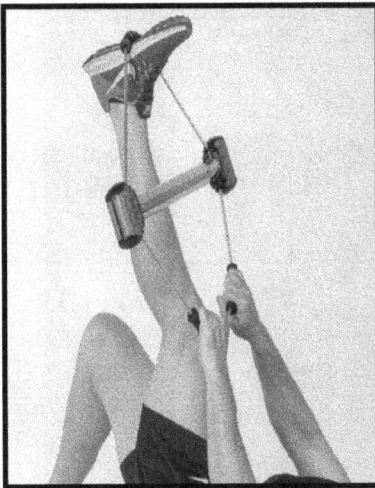

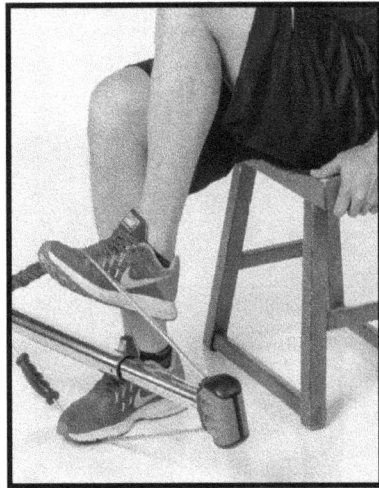

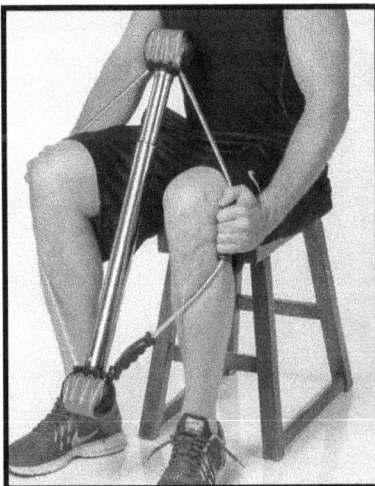

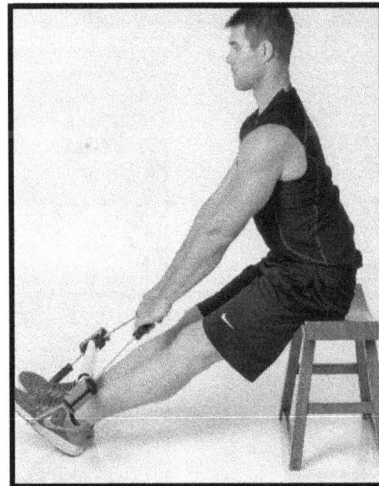

POWER PLUS PROGRAM

06 POWER PLUS STRENGTH PROGRAM

TUESDAY, THURSDAY, SATURDAY
Routine continued...................

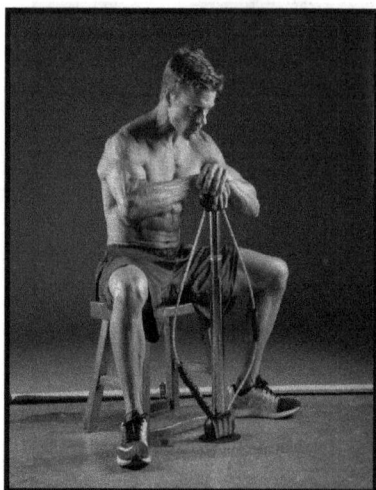

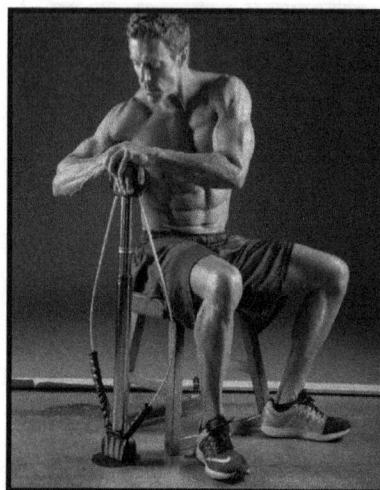

PHASE NINE TUES, THURS, SAT.

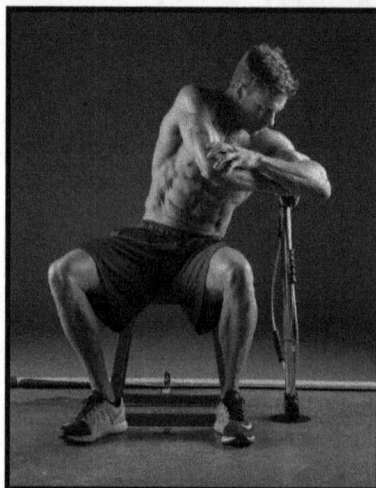

DENSITY POWER RANGE II

07 DENSITY POWER RANGE II PROGRAM 5,8,20

MONDAY, WEDNESDAY, FRIDAY

HOW TO PERFORM THIS ROUTINE: You contract within 1 second and release 2 seconds. Perform 5 reps followed by a 10 second isometric, 8 reps followed by another 10 second isometric, then a final 20 reps. On the 20th rep hold for a 30 second Isometric contraction. **Perform program for 3 weeks**

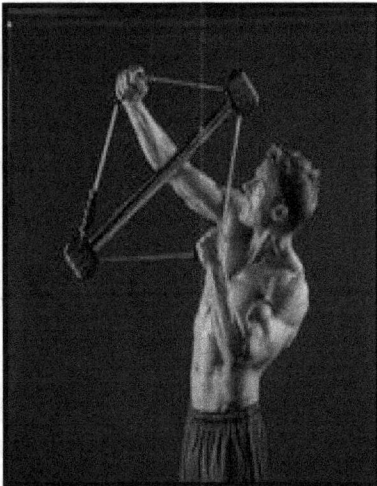

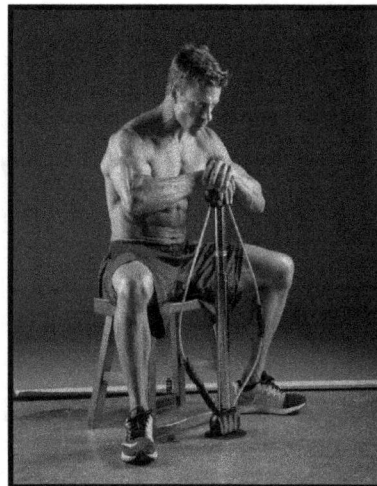

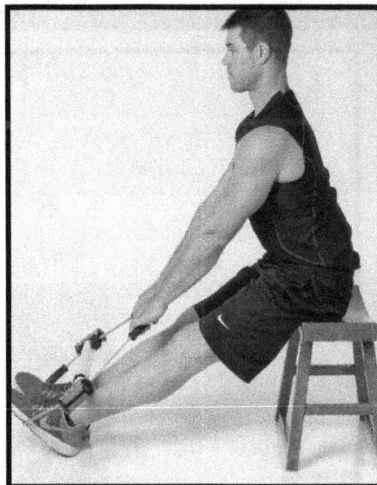

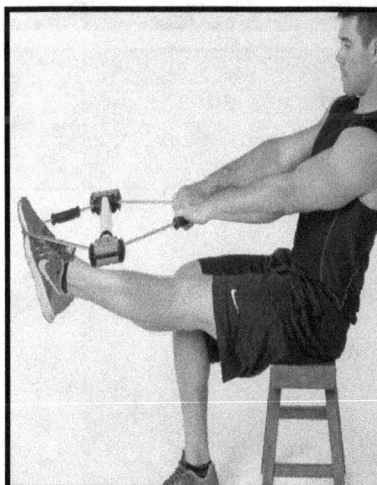

DENSITY POWER RANGE II

07 DENSITY RANGE II PROGRAM 5,8,20

MONDAY, WEDNESDAY, FRIDAY
Routine continued............

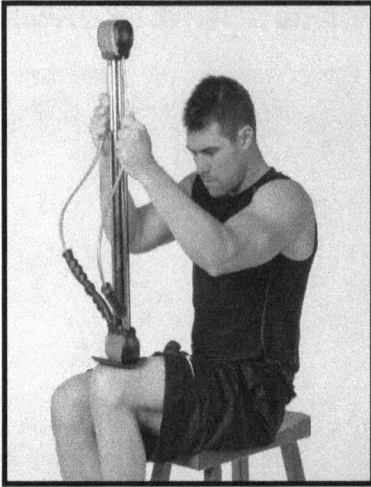

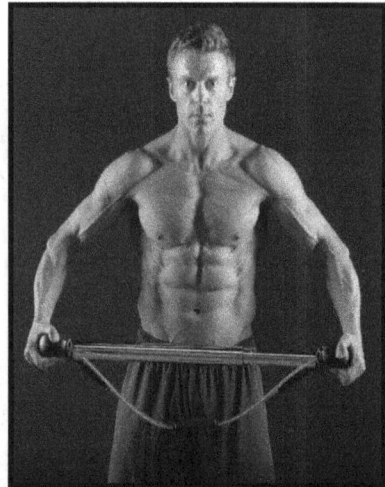

PHASE TEN   MON, WED, FRI.

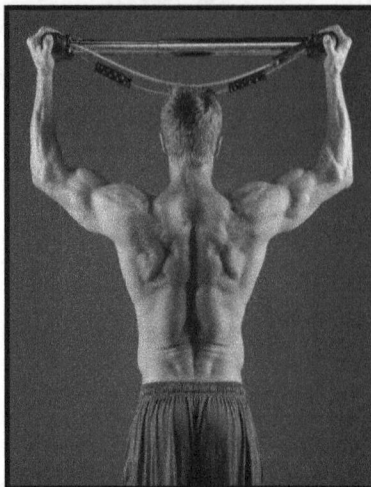

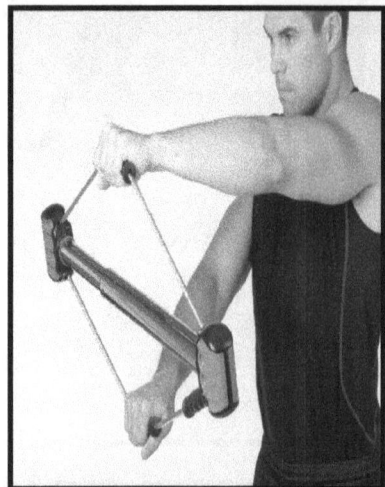

DENSITY POWER MAX II

07 DENSITY POWER MAX II 10,10,10

TUESDAY, THURSDAY, SATURDAY

You contract within 1 second and slowly release the tension for 3 seconds. Perform 10 reps followed by a 20 second isometric, 10 reps followed by another 20 second isometric, then a final 10 reps. On the 10th rep hold for a 7 second Isometric contraction.

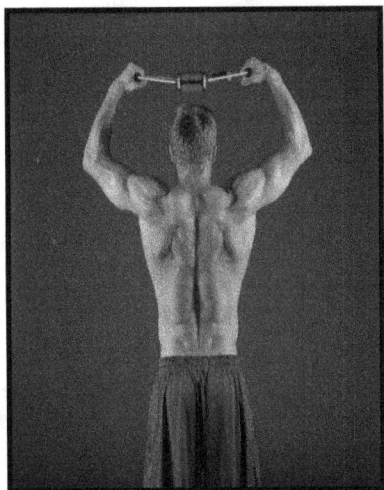

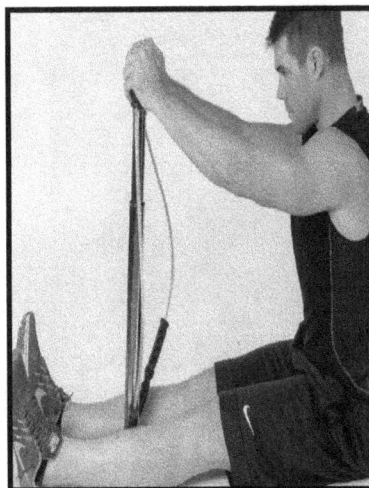

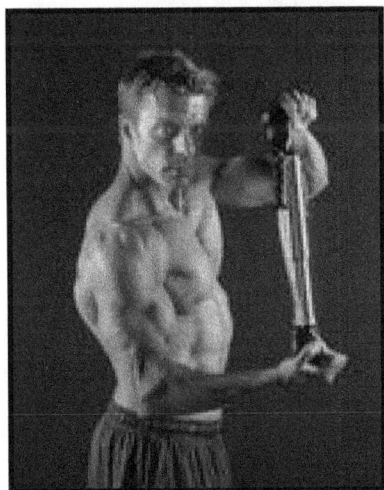

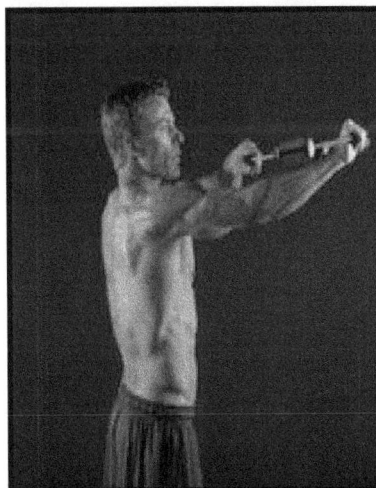

DENSITY POWER MAX II

07 DENSITY POWER MAX II 10,10,10

TUESDAY, THURSDAY, SATURDAY
Routine continued...................

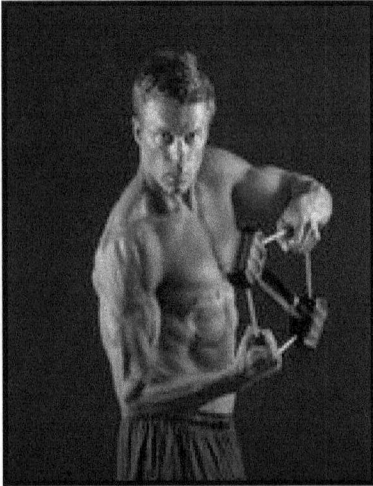

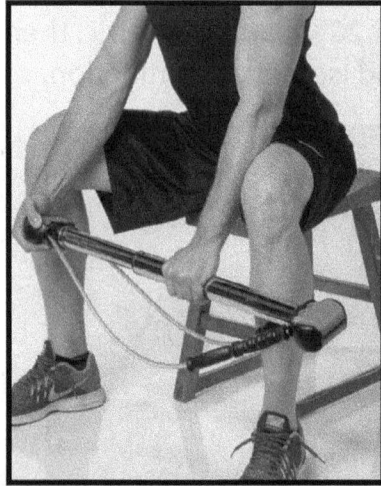

PHASE TEN   TUES, THURS, SAT.

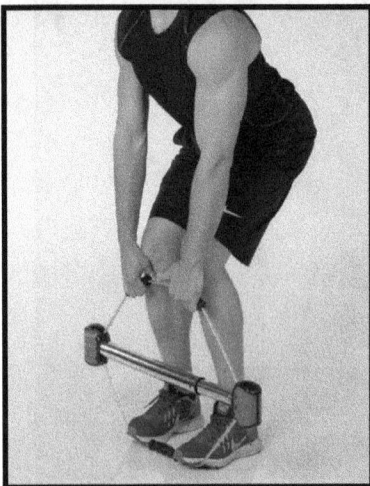

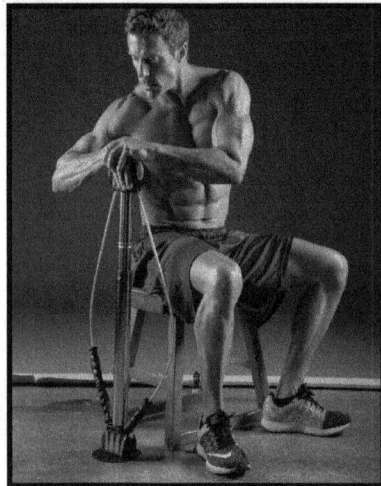

CHAPTER 8
REP RANGE TNT
PHASE 11
2 WEEKS

REP SPEED CONTRACT 1 SECOND, RELEASE 1 SECOND
FIRST WEEK 10 REPS, 20 SECOND ISOMETRIC... 4 ROUNDS
SECOND WEEK 20 REPS, 10 SECOND ISOMETRIC.. 4 ROUNDS
THIRD WEEK 30 REPS, 20 SECOND ISOMETRIC... 4 ROUNDS

REP RANGE TNT

08 REP RANGE TNT PROGRAM

HOW TO PERFORM THIS ROUTINE:
First Week: 10 reps, 20 second Isometric contraction 4 rounds.
Second Week: 20 reps, 10 second Isometric contraction 4 rounds.
Third Week: 30 reps, 20 second Isometric contraction 4 rounds.

DAY ONE

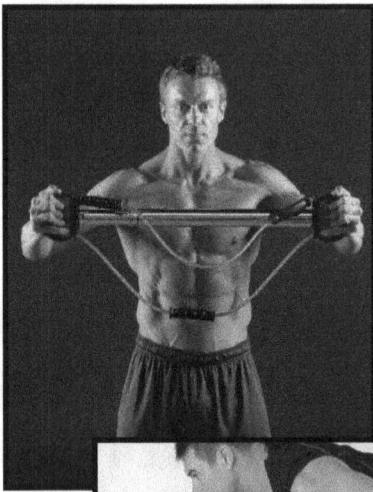
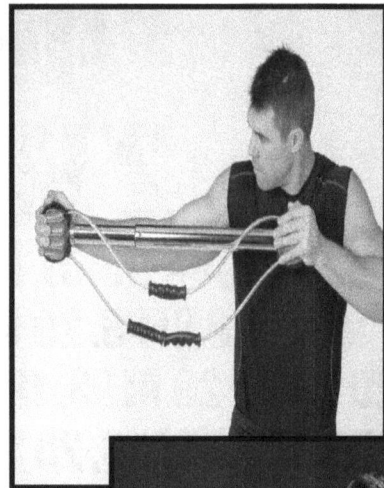
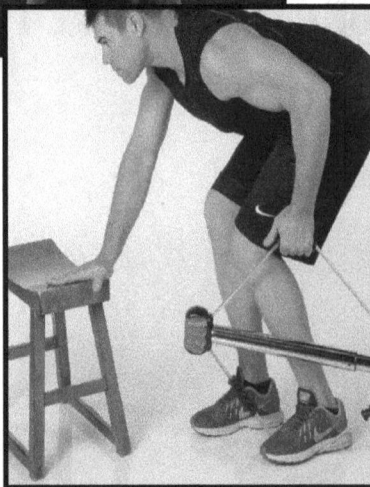
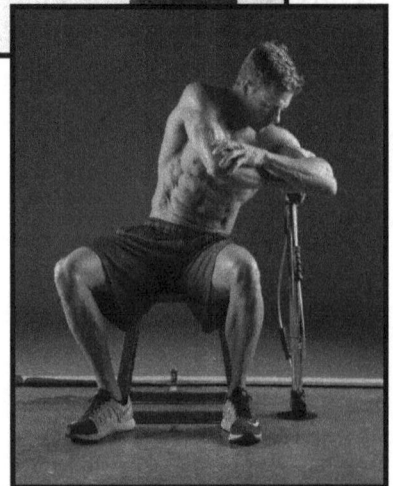

REP RANGE TNT

08 REP RANGE TNT PROGRAM

HOW TO PERFORM THIS ROUTINE:
First Week: 10 reps, 20 second Isometric contraction 4 rounds.
Second Week: 20 reps, 10 second Isometric contraction 4 rounds.
Third Week: 30 reps, 20 second Isometric contraction 4 rounds.

DAY ONE continued.........

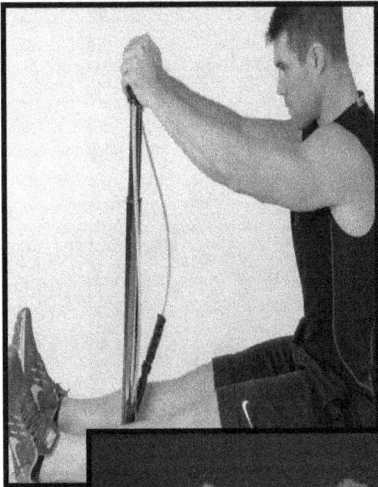

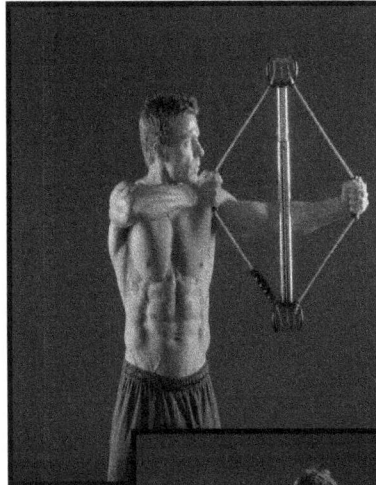

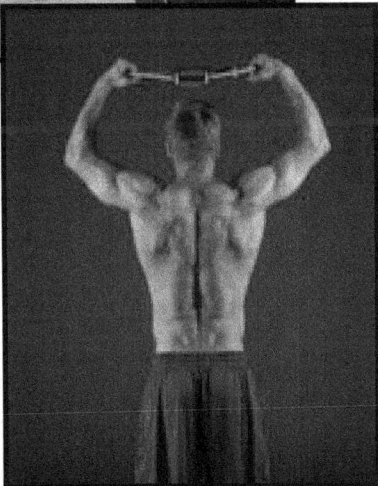

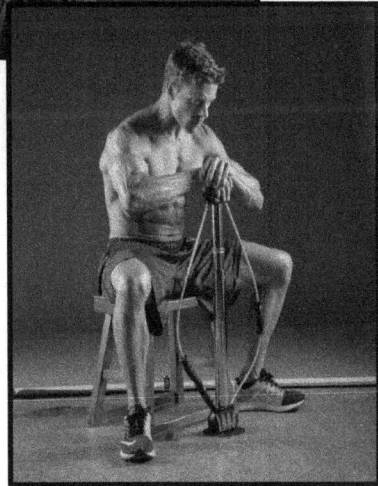

REP RANGE TNT

08 REP RANGE TNT PROGRAM

HOW TO PERFORM THIS ROUTINE:
First Week: 10 reps, 20 second Isometric contraction 4 rounds.
Second Week: 20 reps, 10 second Isometric contraction 4 rounds.
Third Week: 30 reps, 20 second Isometric contraction 4 rounds.

DAY TWO

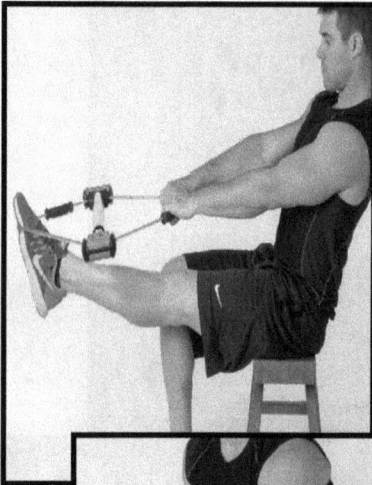
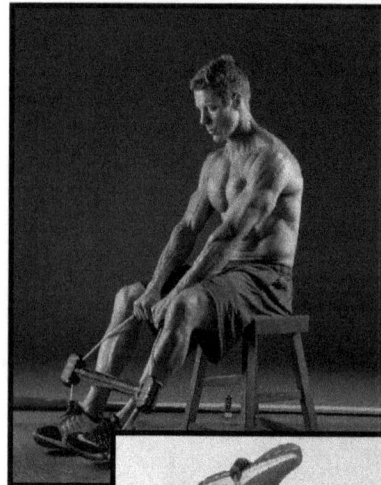
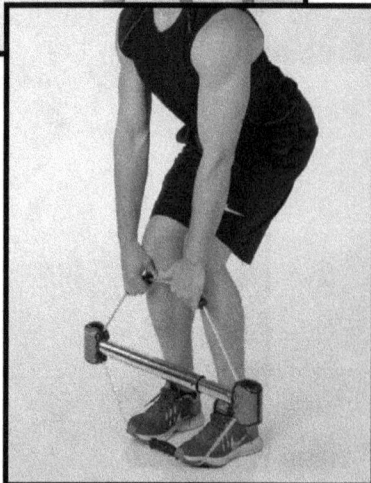
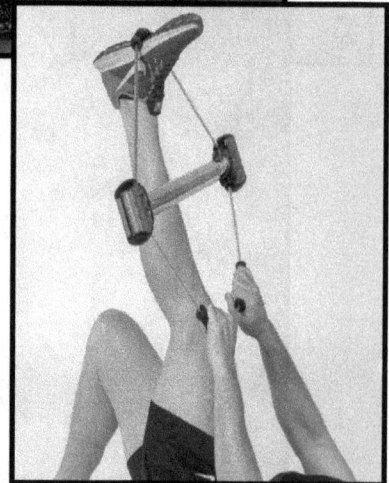

REP RANGE TNT

08 REP RANGE TNT PROGRAM

HOW TO PERFORM THIS ROUTINE:
First Week: 10 reps, 20 second Isometric contraction 4 rounds.
Second Week: 20 reps, 10 second Isometric contraction 4 rounds.
Third Week: 30 reps, 20 second Isometric contraction 4 rounds.

DAY TWO continued............

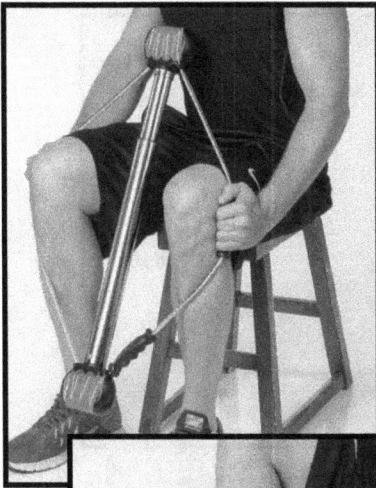

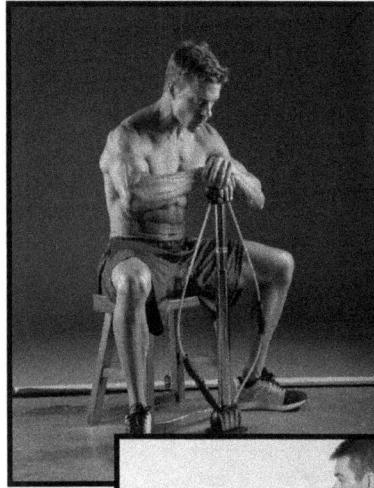

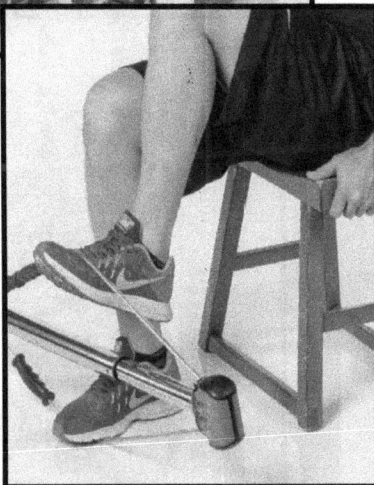

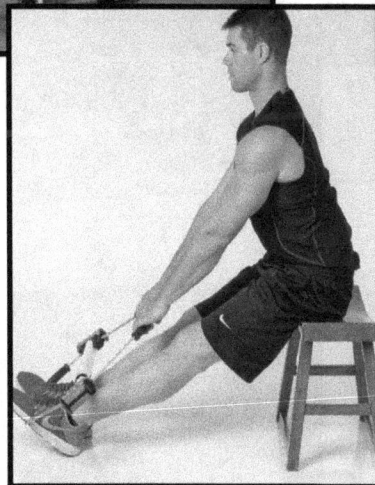

REP RANGE TNT

08 REP RANGE TNT PROGRAM

HOW TO PERFORM THIS ROUTINE:
First Week: 10 reps, 20 second Isometric contraction 4 rounds.
Second Week: 20 reps, 10 second Isometric contraction 4 rounds.
Third Week: 30 reps, 20 second Isometric contraction 4 rounds.

DAY THREE

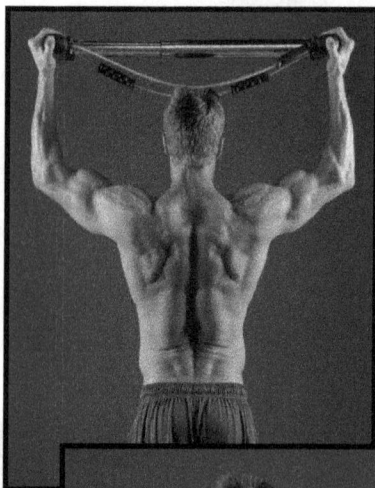
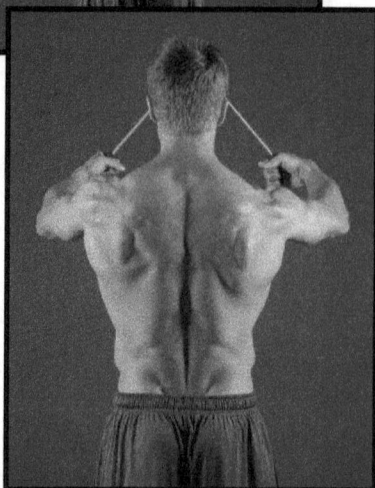
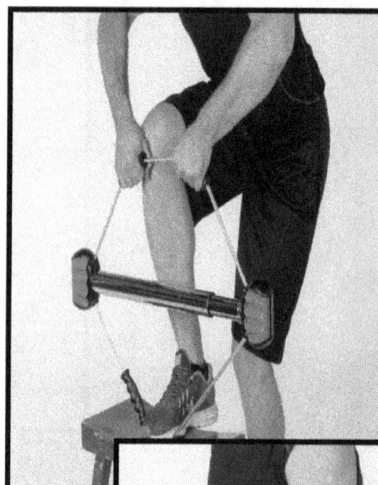
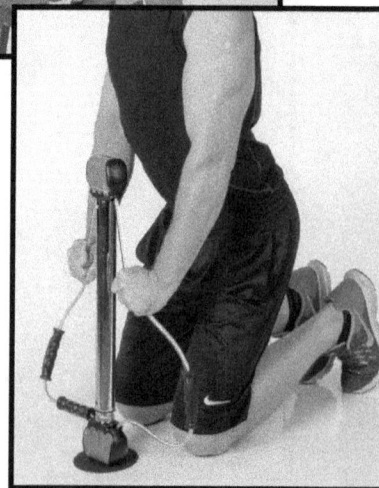

REP RANGE TNT

08 REP RANGE TNT PROGRAM

HOW TO PERFORM THIS ROUTINE:
First Week: 10 reps, 20 second Isometric contraction 4 rounds.
Second Week: 20 reps, 10 second Isometric contraction 4 rounds.
Third Week: 30 reps, 20 second Isometric contraction 4 rounds.

DAY THREE continued.......

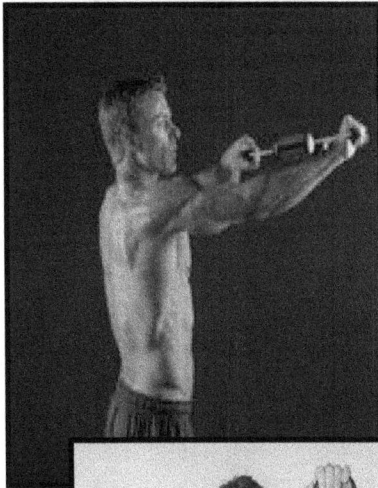

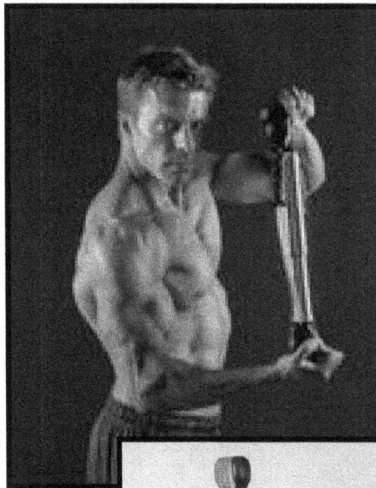

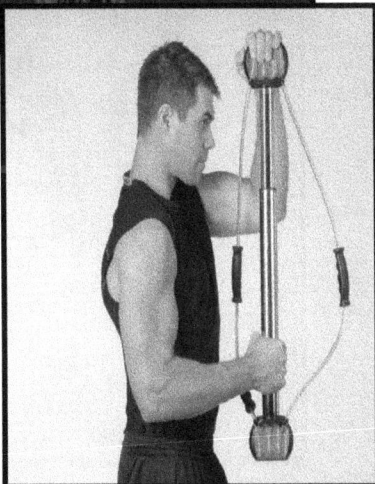

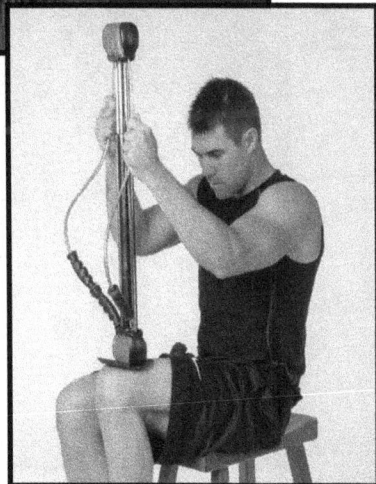

REP RANGE TNT

08 REP RANGE TNT PROGRAM

HOW TO PERFORM THIS ROUTINE:
First Week: 10 reps, 20 second Isometric contraction 4 rounds.
Second Week: 20 reps, 10 second Isometric contraction 4 rounds.
Third Week: 30 reps, 20 second Isometric contraction 4 rounds.

DAY THREE continued.......

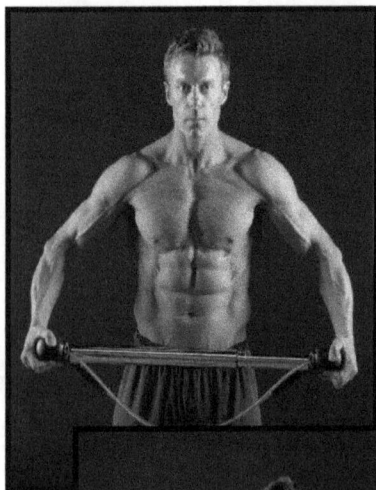

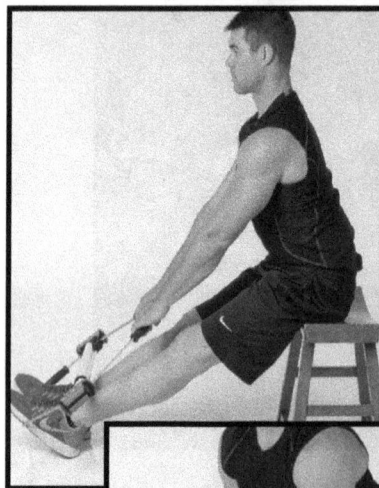

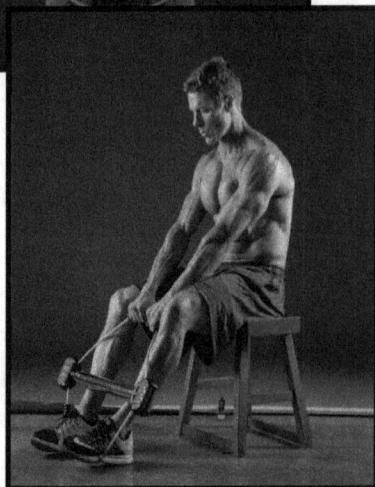

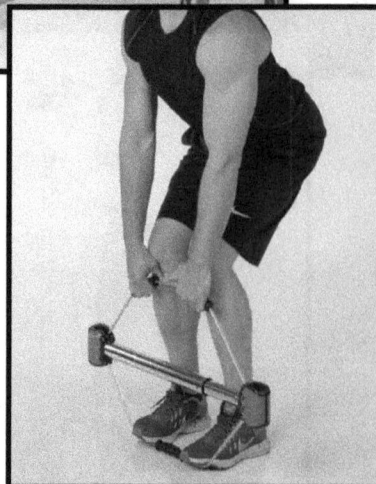

REP RANGE TNT

08 REP RANGE TNT PROGRAM

HOW TO PERFORM THIS ROUTINE:
First Week: 10 reps, 20 second Isometric contraction 4 rounds.
Second Week: 20 reps, 10 second Isometric contraction 4 rounds.
Third Week: 30 reps, 20 second Isometric contraction 4 rounds.

DAY FOUR

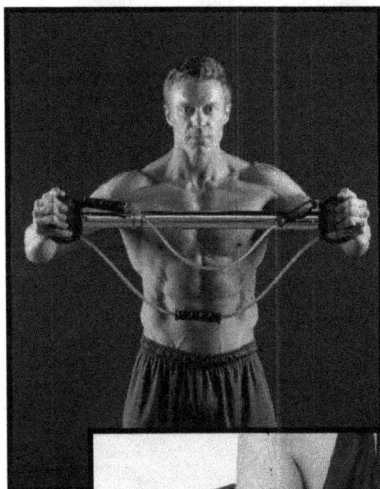
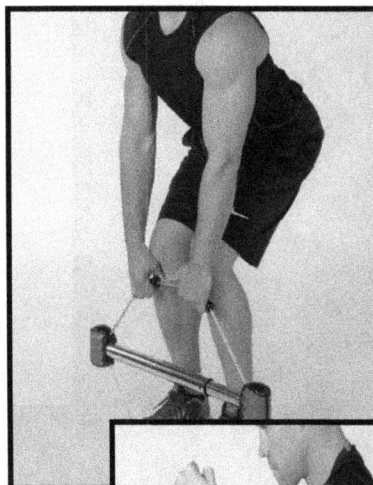
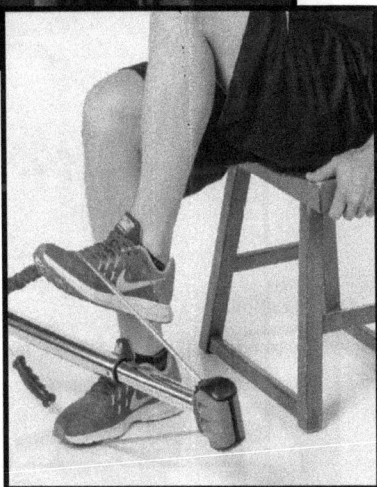
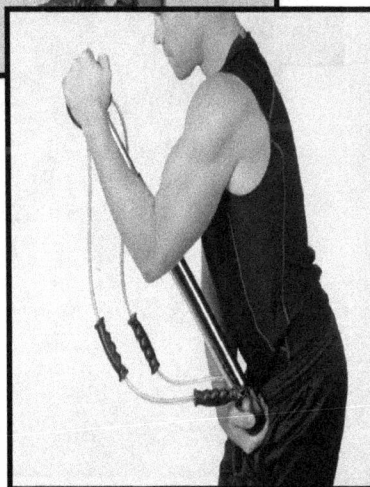

REP RANGE TNT

08 REP RANGE TNT PROGRAM

HOW TO PERFORM THIS ROUTINE:
First Week: 10 reps, 20 second Isometric contraction 4 rounds.
Second Week: 20 reps, 10 second Isometric contraction 4 rounds.
Third Week: 30 reps, 30 second Isometric contraction 4 rounds.

DAY FOUR continued......

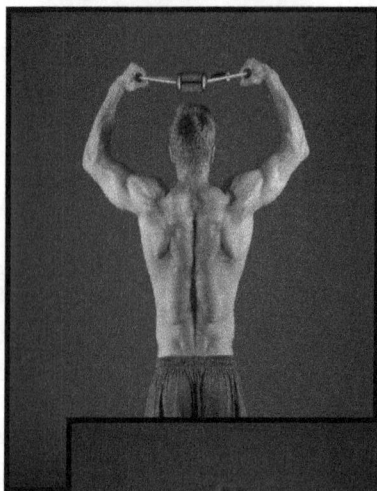

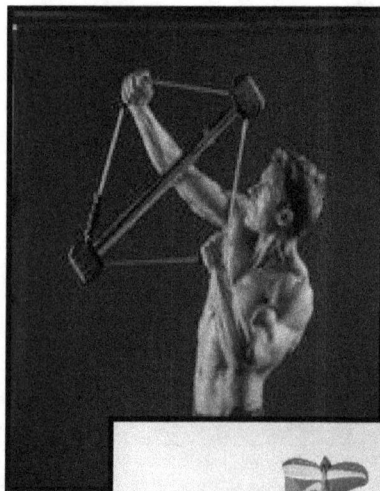

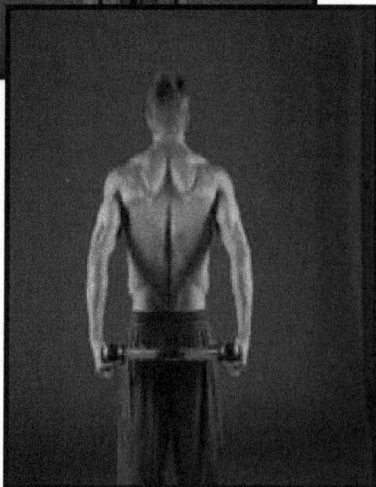

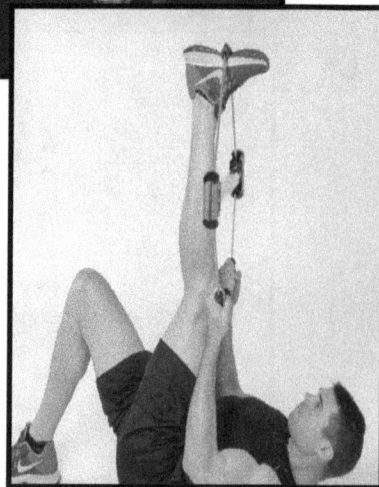

REP RANGE TNT

08 REP RANGE TNT PROGRAM

HOW TO PERFORM THIS ROUTINE:
First Week: 10 reps, 20 second Isometric contraction 4 rounds.
Second Week: 20 reps, 10 second Isometric contraction 4 rounds.
Third Week: 30 reps, 20 second Isometric contraction 4 rounds.

DAY FIVE

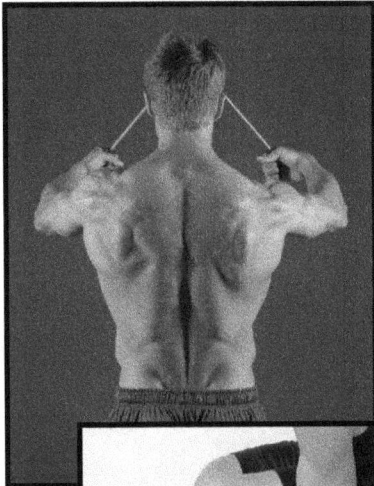
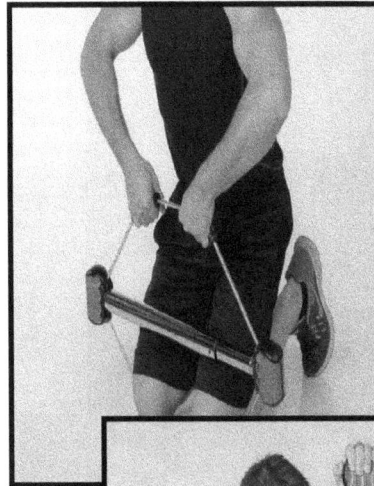
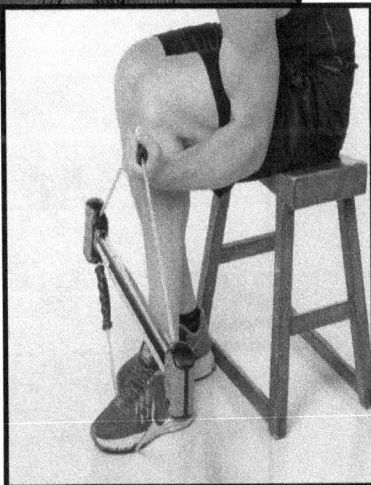
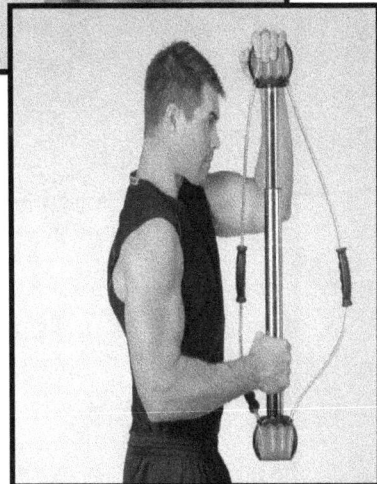

REP RANGE TNT

08 REP RANGE TNT PROGRAM

HOW TO PERFORM THIS ROUTINE:
First Week: 10 reps, 20 second Isometric contraction 4 rounds.
Second Week: 20 reps, 10 second Isometric contraction 4 rounds.
Third Week: 30 reps, 20 second Isometric contraction 4 rounds.

DAY FIVE continued.....

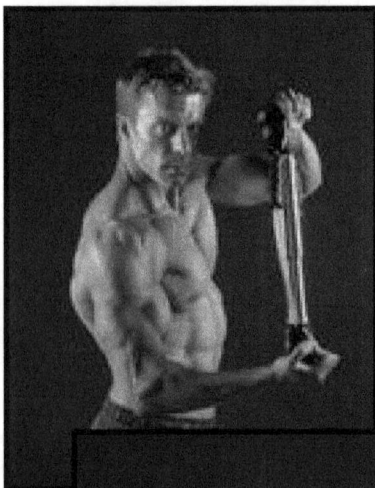
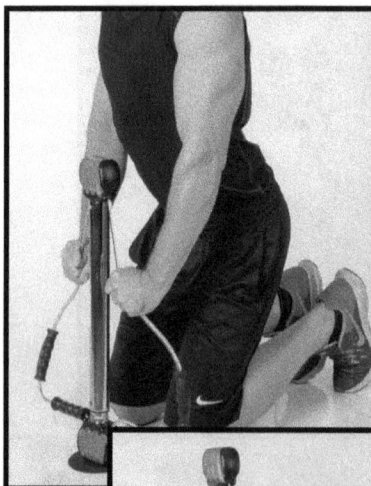
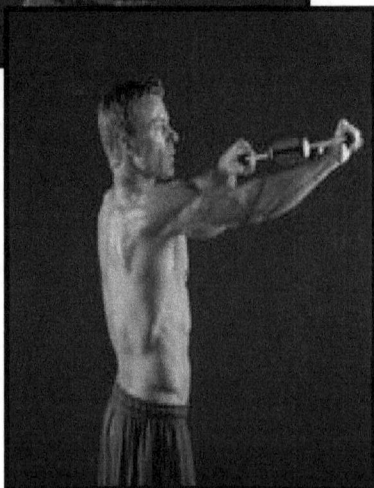
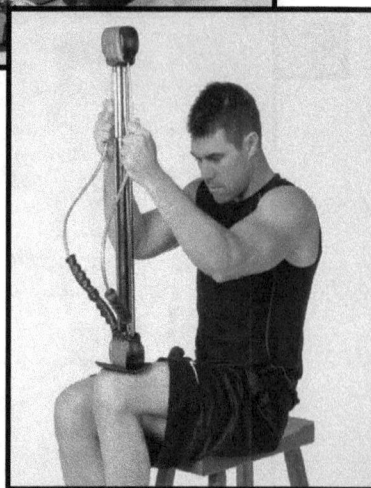

CHAPTER 9
REP RANGE II
POWER PUMP 30
PHASE 1
WEEK 1 OF 3
REP SPEED CONTRACT 1 SECOND, RELEASE 2 SECONDS

REP RANGE POWER PUMP 30 PROGRAM

09 REP RANGE POWER PUMP 30 PROGRAM

REP RANGE POWER PUMP 30 PROGRAM " MUSCLE-BUILDING PHASE"

Phase 1: 30x20 Perform 30 reps followed by a 20 second isometric contraction. 3 sets per exercise

Phase 2: 30x30 Perform 30 reps followed by a 30 second isometric contraction. 3 sets per exercise.

Phase 3: 30x20 Perform 15 reps followed by a 20 second isometric contraction. 3 set per exercise

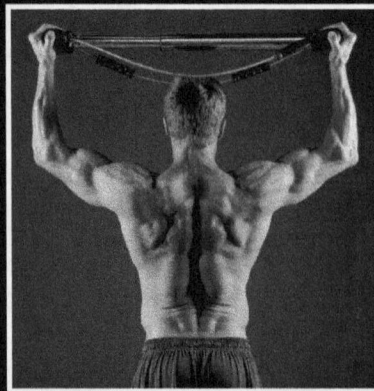

PHASE ONE 30X20

09 REP RANGE POWER PUMP 30 PROGRAM

HOW TO PERFORM THIS ROUTINE:
PHASE ONE 20x10 PHASE

Perform 30 reps followed by a 20 second isometric contraction.
3 sets per exercise

DAY ONE

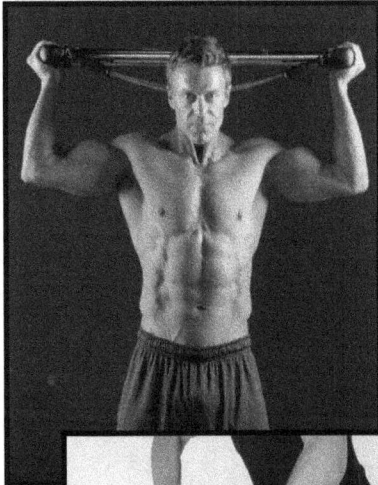

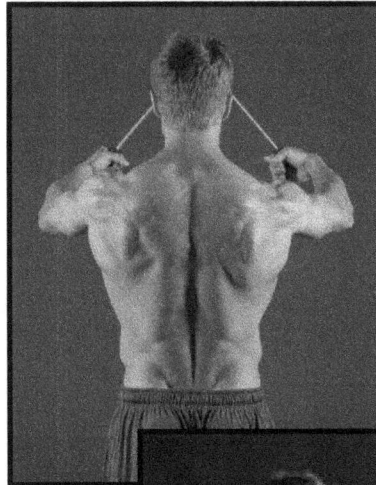

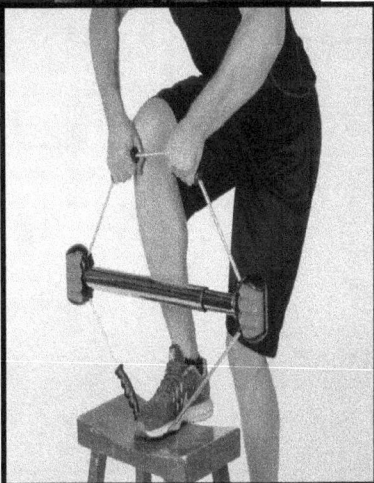

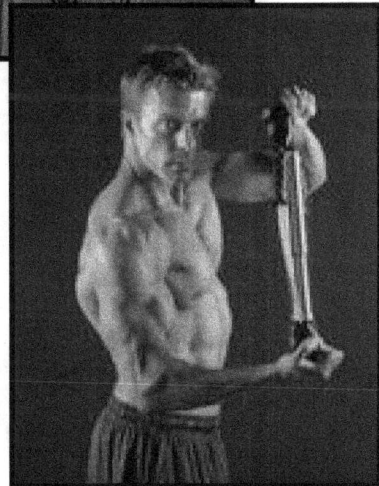

PHASE ONE 30X20

09 REP RANGE POWER PUMP 30 PROGRAM

HOW TO PERFORM THIS ROUTINE:
PHASE ONE 30x20 PHASE

Perform 30 reps followed by a 20 second isometric contraction.
3 sets per exercise

DAY ONE continued............

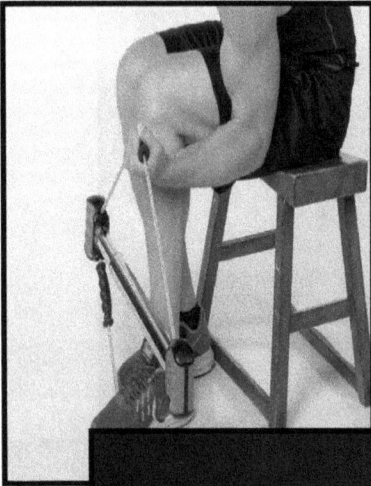

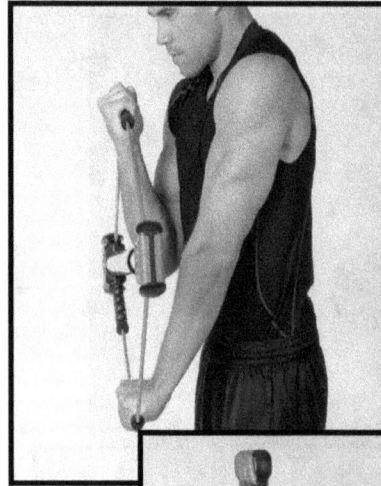

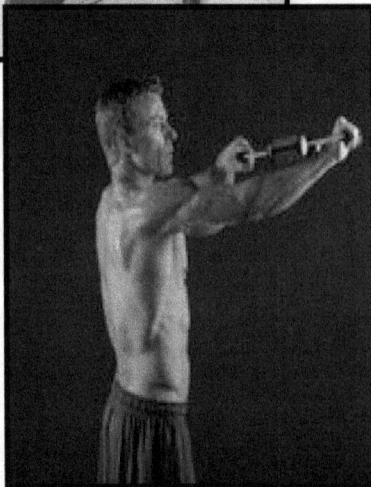

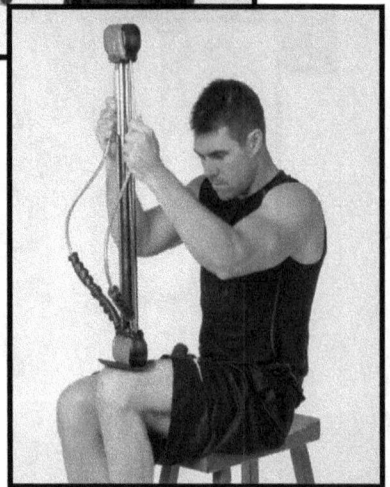

PHASE ONE 30X20

09 REP RANGE POWER PUMP 30 PROGRAM

HOW TO PERFORM THIS ROUTINE:
PHASE ONE 30x20 PHASE

Perform 30 reps followed by a 20 second isometric contraction.
3 sets per exercise

DAY TWO

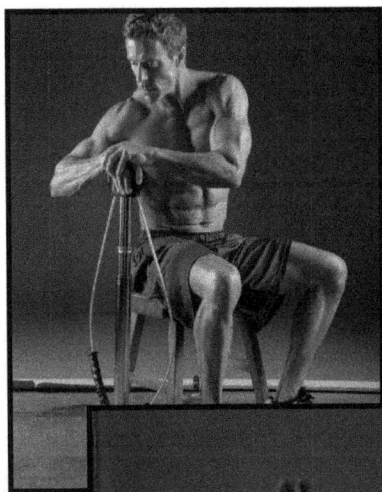
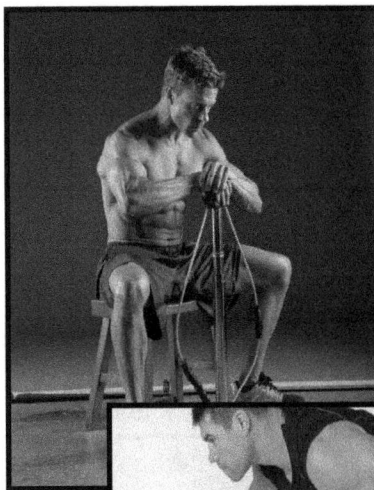
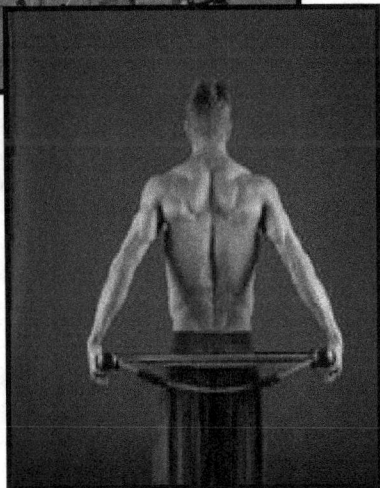
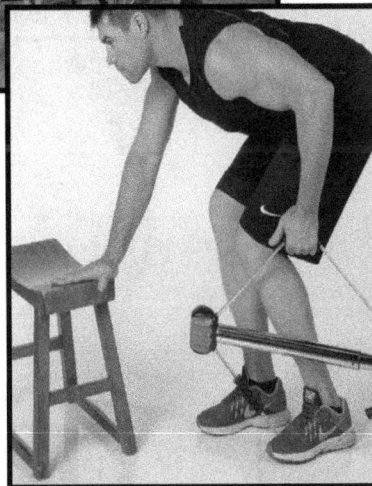

PHASE ONE 30X20

09 REP RANGE POWER MAX 20 PROGRAM

HOW TO PERFORM THIS ROUTINE:
PHASE ONE 30x20 PHASE
Perform 30 reps followed by a 20 second isometric contraction.
3 sets per exercise

DAY TWO continued.......

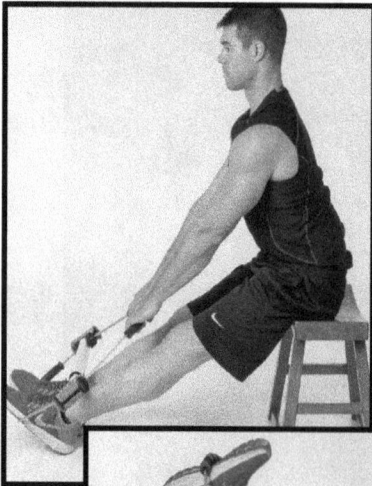

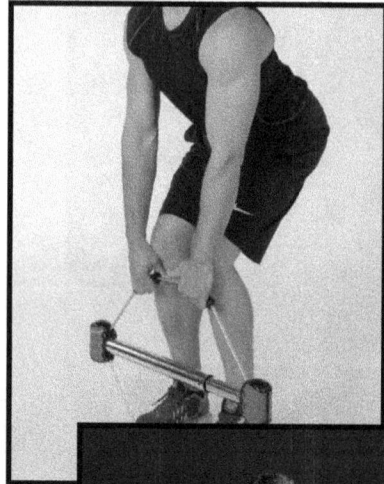

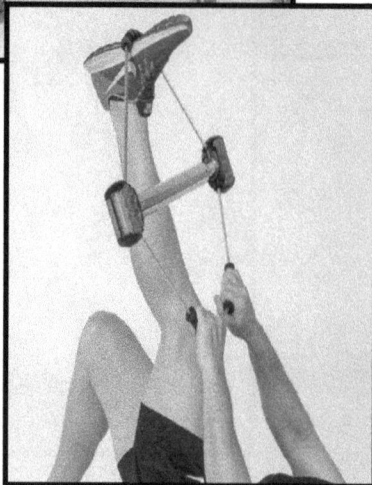

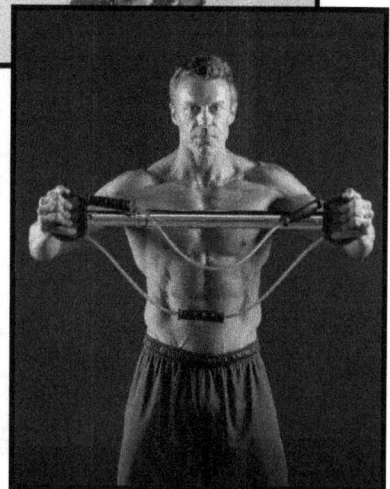

PHASE ONE 30X20

09 REP RANGE POWER PUMP 30 PROGRAM

HOW TO PERFORM THIS ROUTINE:
PHASE ONE 30x20 PHASE
Perform 30 reps followed by a 20 second isometric contraction.
3 sets per exercise

DAY THREE

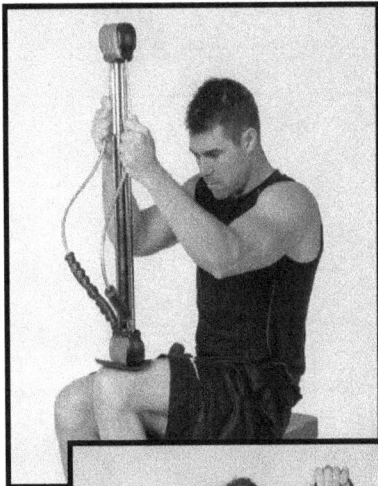
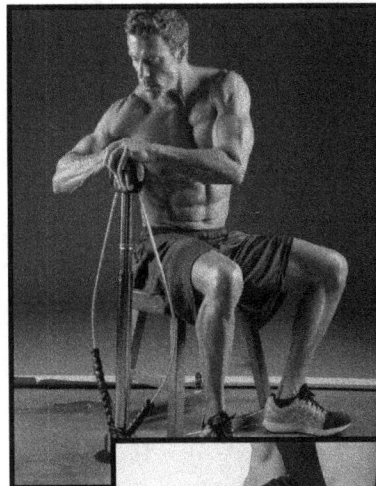
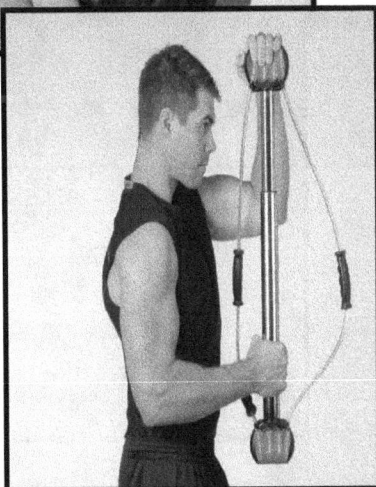
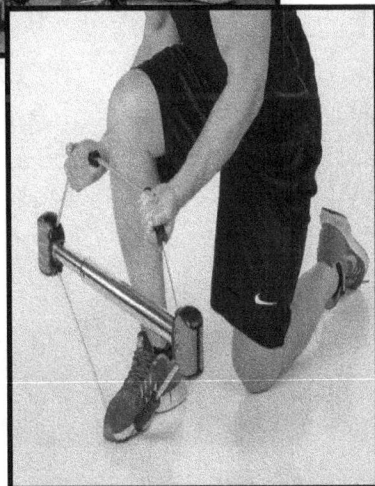

PHASE ONE 30X20

09 REP RANGE POWER PUMP 30 PROGRAM

HOW TO PERFORM THIS ROUTINE:
PHASE ONE 30x20 PHASE

Perform 30 reps followed by a 20 second isometric contraction.
3 sets per exercise

DAY THREE continued..........

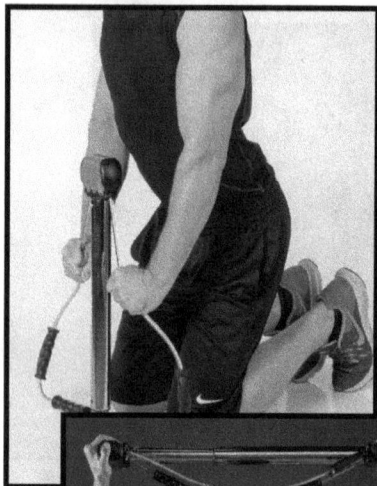
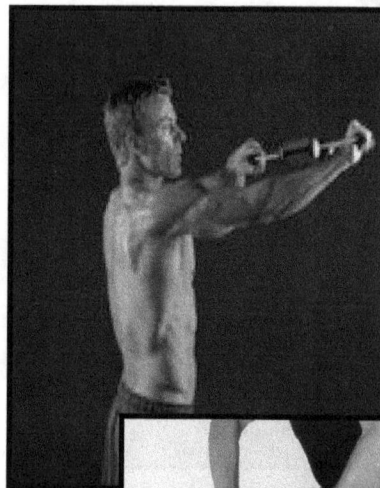
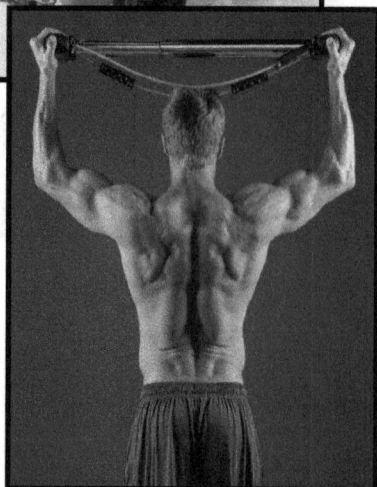
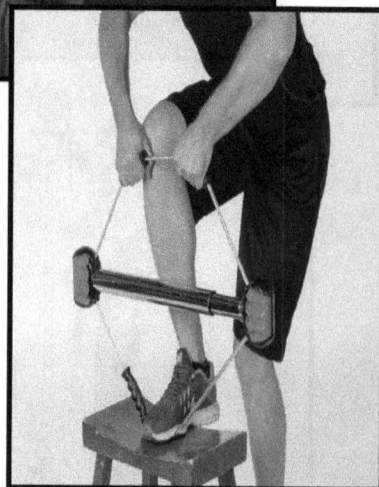

PHASE ONE 30X20

09 REP RANGE POWER PUMP 30 PROGRAM

HOW TO PERFORM THIS ROUTINE:
PHASE ONE 30x20 PHASE

Perform 30 reps followed by a 20 second isometric contraction.
3 sets per exercise

DAY FOUR

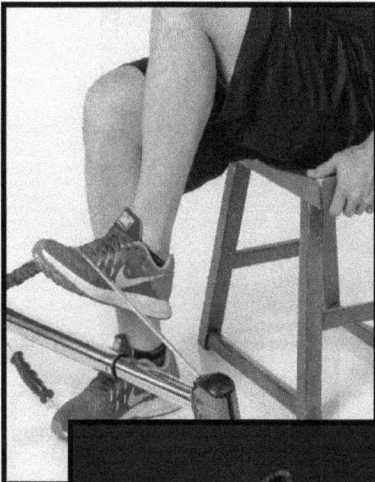

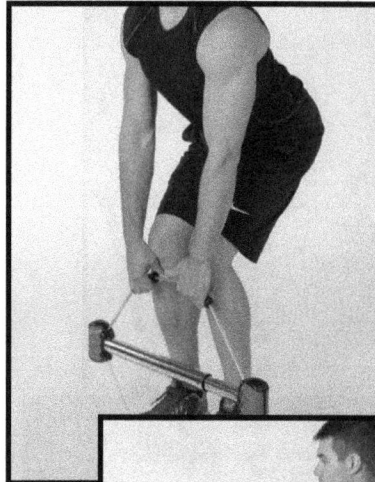

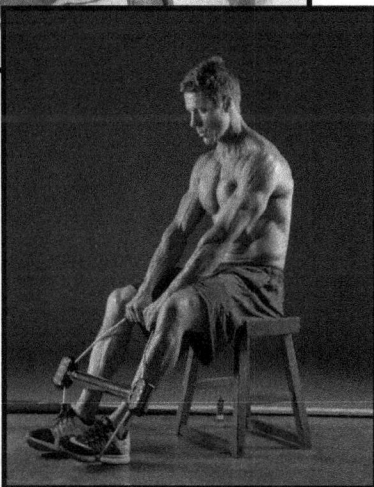

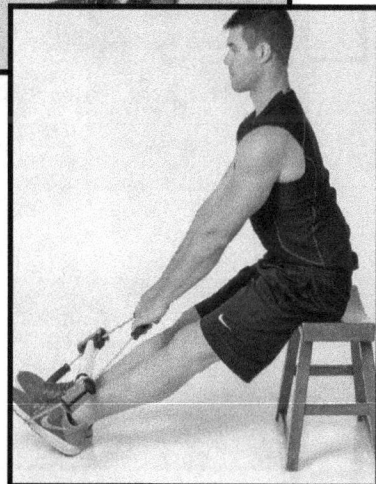

PHASE ONE 30X20

09 REP RANGE POWER PUMP 30 PROGRAM

HOW TO PERFORM THIS ROUTINE:
PHASE ONE 30x20 PHASE

Perform 30 reps followed by a 20 second isometric contraction.
3 sets per exercise

DAY FOUR continued...........

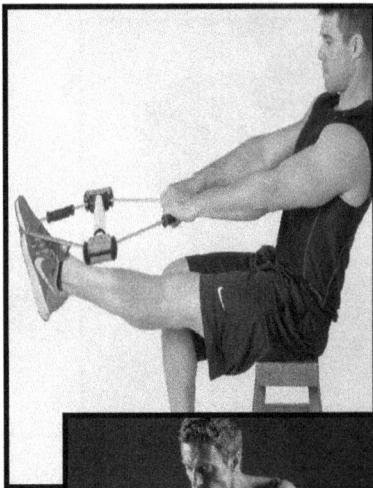

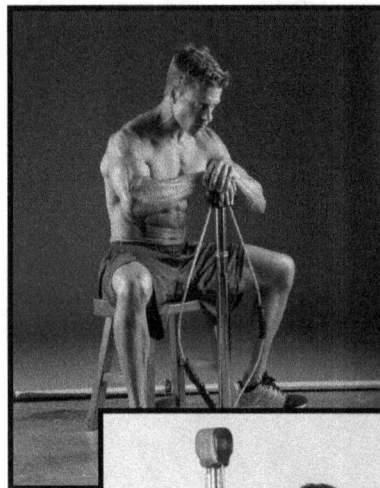

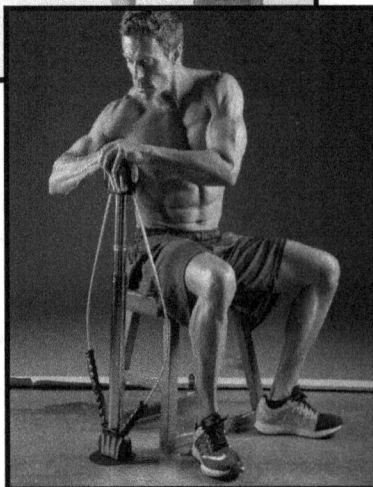

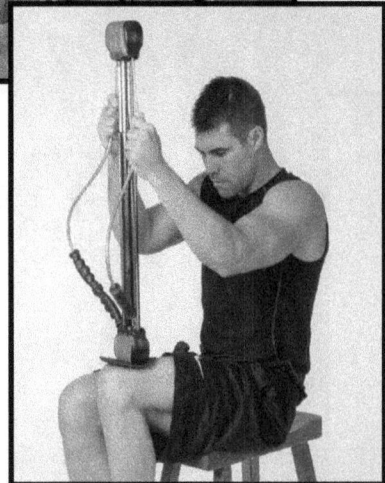

PHASE ONE 30X20

09 REP RANGE POWER PUMP 30 PROGRAM

HOW TO PERFORM THIS ROUTINE:
PHASE ONE 30x20 PHASE

Perform 30 reps followed by a 20 second isometric contraction.
3 sets per exercise

DAY FIVE

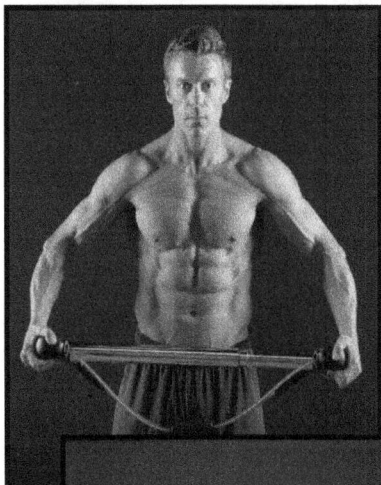

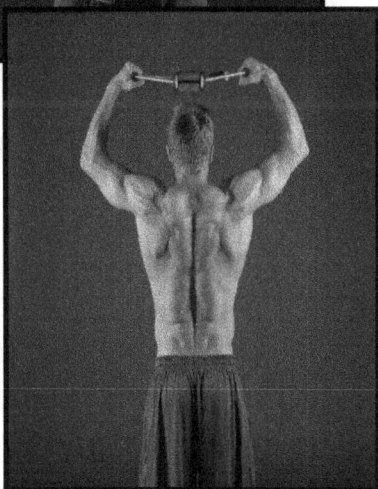

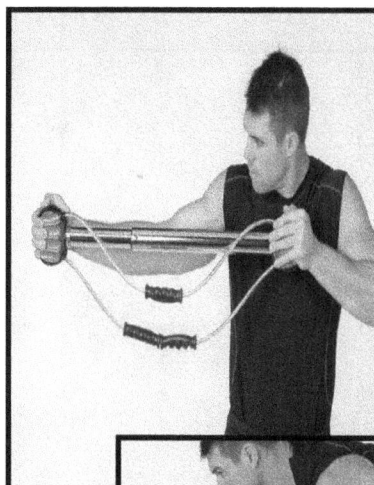

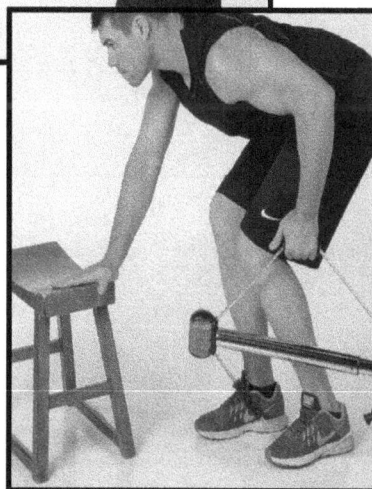

PHASE ONE 30X20

09 REP RANGE POWER PUMP 30 PROGRAM

HOW TO PERFORM THIS ROUTINE:
PHASE ONE 30x20 PHASE

Perform 30 reps followed by a 20 second isometric contraction.
3 sets per exercise

DAY FIVE continued.............

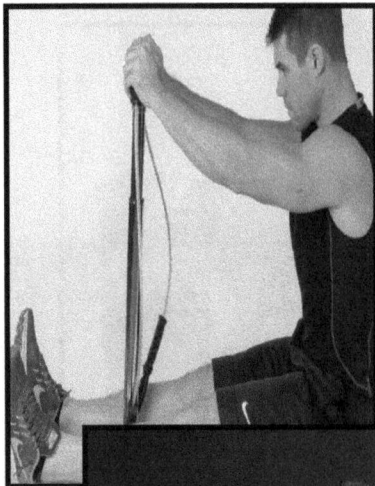

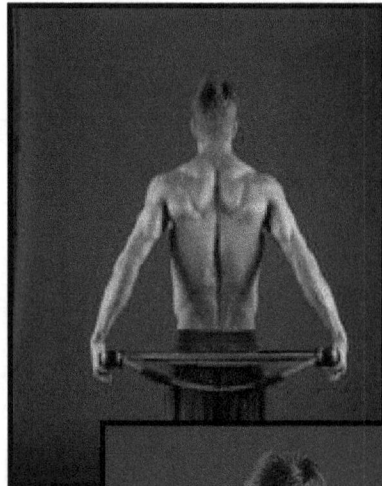

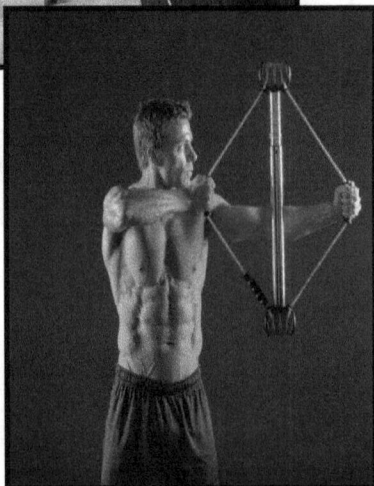

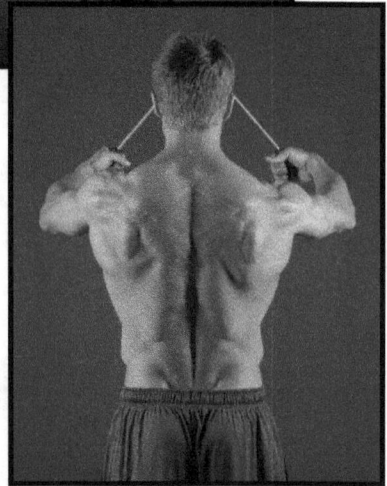

CHAPTER 9
REP RANGE II
POWER PUMP 30
PHASE 2
WEEK 2 OF 3
REP SPEED CONTRACT 2 SECOND, RELEASE 2 SECOND, ALTERNATE DAY ONE AND DAY TWO FOR 6 DAYS OF TRAINING

PHASE TWO 30X30

09 REP RANGE POWER PUMP 30 PROGRAM

HOW TO PERFORM THIS ROUTINE:
PHASE TWO 30x30 PHASE
Perform 30 reps followed by a 30 second isometric contraction.
3 sets per exercise

DAY ONE

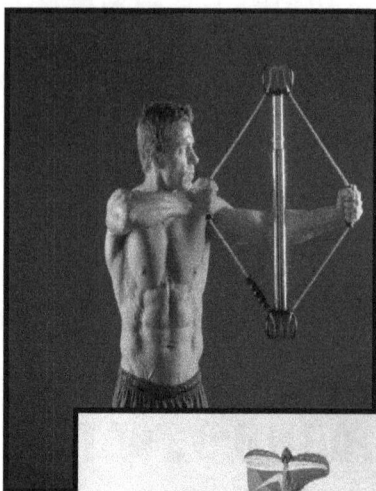
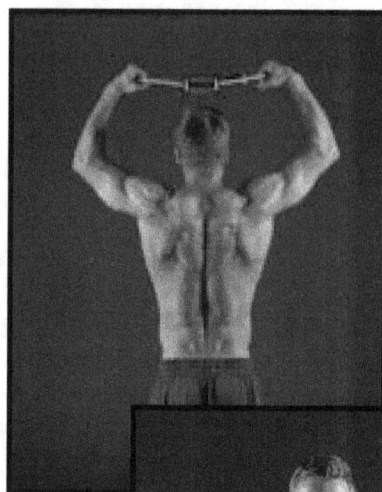
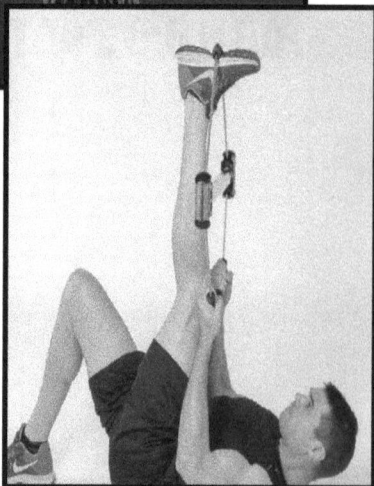
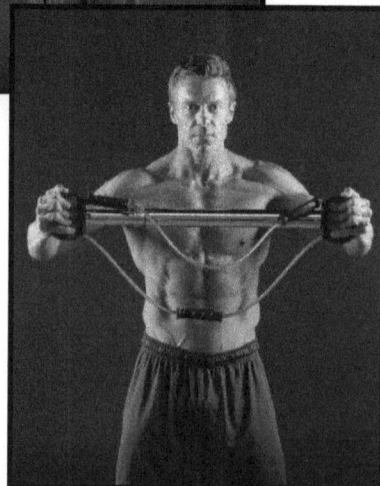

PHASE TWO 30X30

09 REP RANGE POWER PUMP 30 PROGRAM

HOW TO PERFORM THIS ROUTINE:
PHASE TWO 30x30 PHASE
Perform 30 reps followed by a 30 second isometric contraction.
3 sets per exercise

DAY ONE continued..........

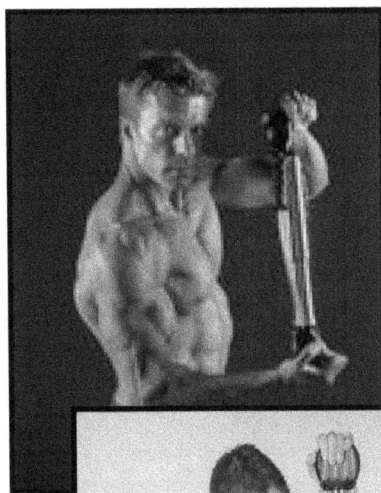

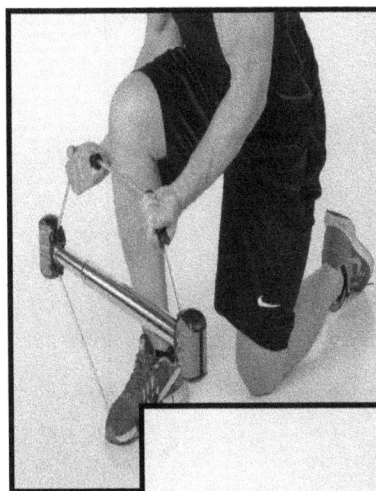

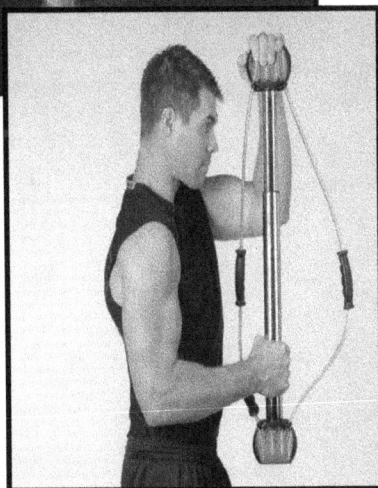

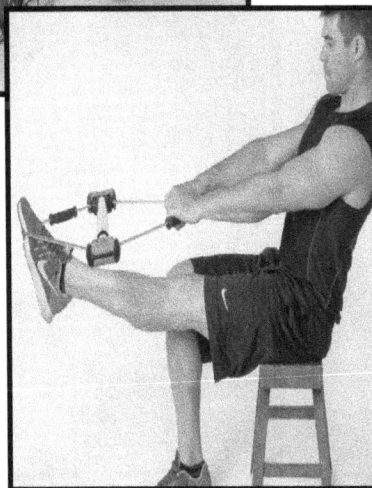

PHASE TWO 30X30

09 REP RANGE POWER PUMP 30 PROGRAM

HOW TO PERFORM THIS ROUTINE:
PHASE TWO 30x30 PHASE

Perform 30 reps followed by a 30 second isometric contraction.
3 sets per exercise

DAY TWO

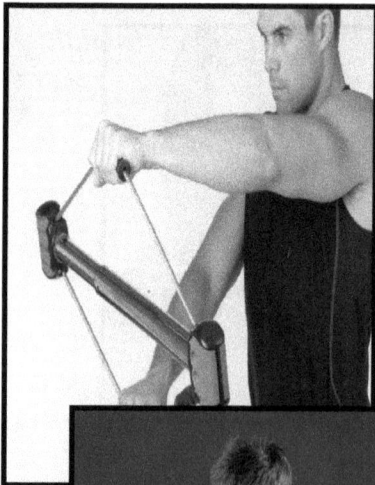
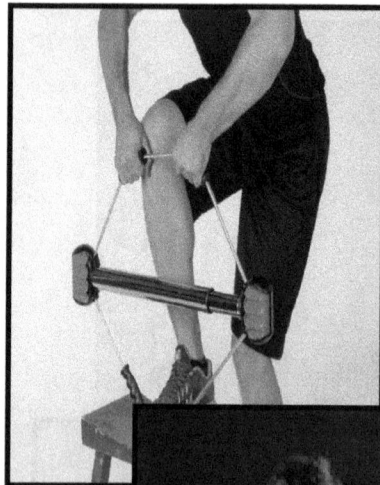
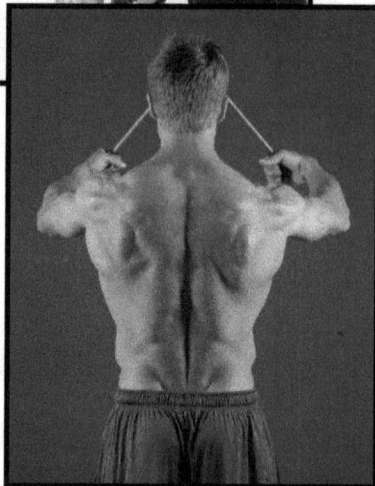
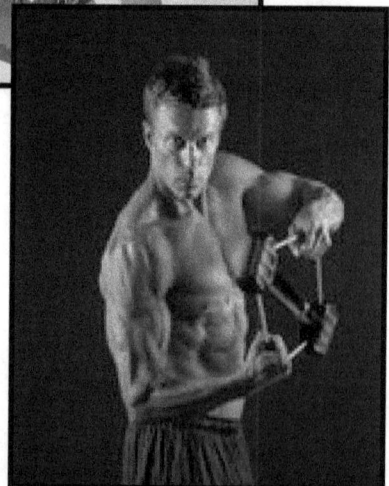

PHASE TWO 30X30

09 REP RANGE POWER PUMP 30 PROGRAM

HOW TO PERFORM THIS ROUTINE:
PHASE TWO 30x30 PHASE
Perform 30 reps followed by a 30 second isometric contraction.
3 sets per exercise

DAY TWO continued........

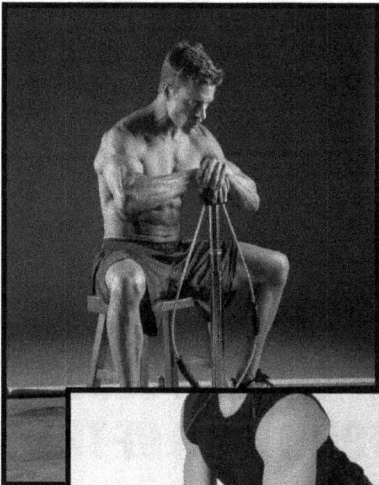

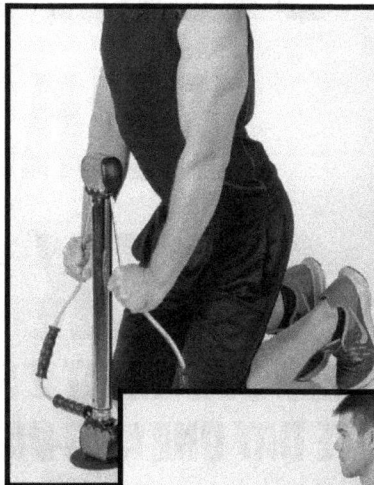

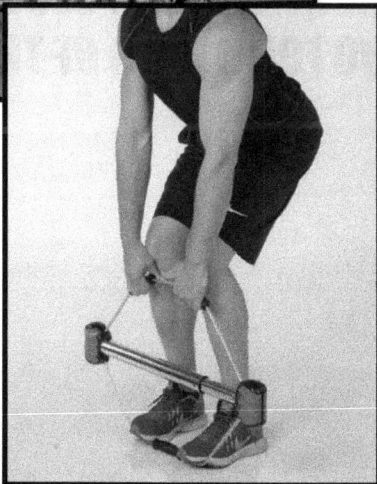

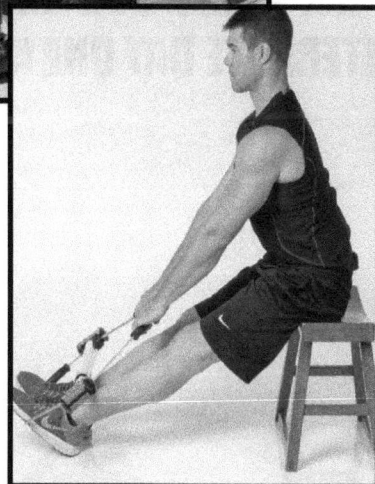

CHAPTER 9

REP RANGE II

POWER PUMP 30

PHASE 3

WEEK 3 OF 3

REP SPEED CONTRACT 2 SECOND, RELEASE 2 SECOND, ALTERNATE DAY ONE AND DAY TWO FOR 6 DAYS OF TRAINING

PHASE THREE 30X20

09 REP RANGE POWER PUMP 30 PROGRAM

HOW TO PERFORM THIS ROUTINE:
PHASE TWO 30x20 PHASE

Perform 30 reps followed by a 20 second isometric contraction.
3 sets per exercise

DAY ONE

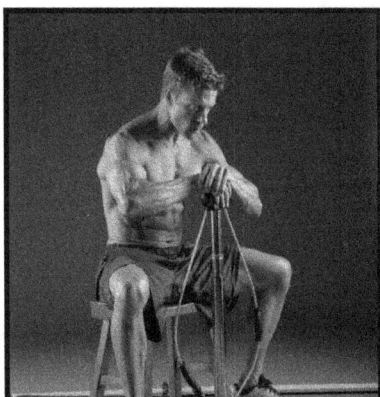
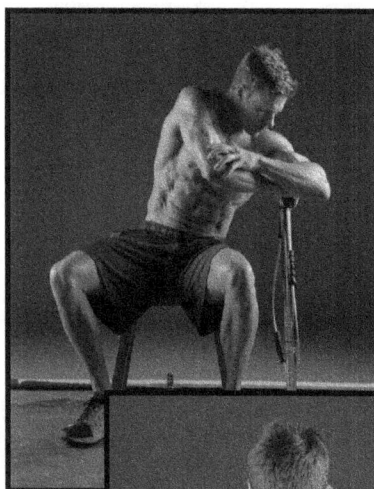
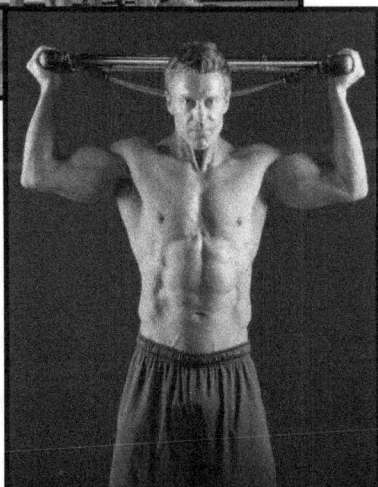
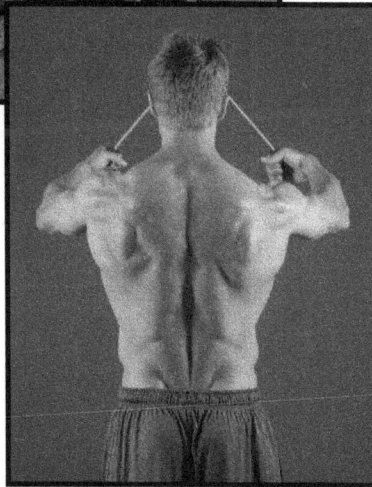

PHASE THREE 30X20

09 REP RANGE POWER PUMP 30 PROGRAM

HOW TO PERFORM THIS ROUTINE:
PHASE TWO 30x20 PHASE
Perform 30 reps followed by a 20 second isometric contraction.
3 sets per exercise

DAY ONE continued...........

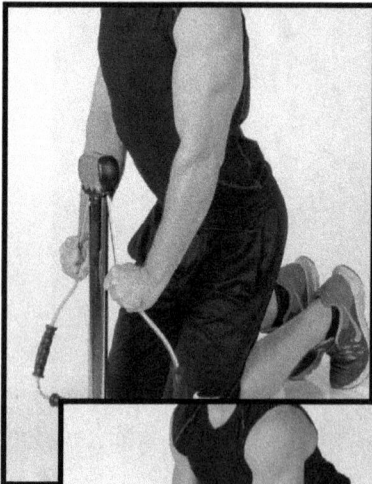

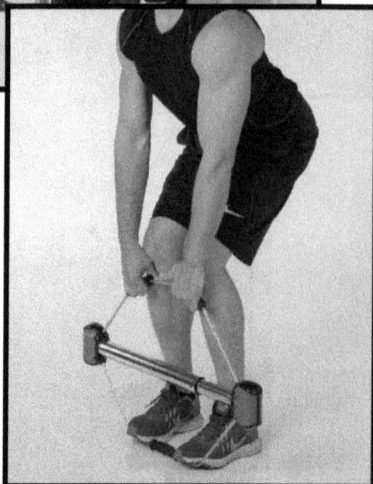

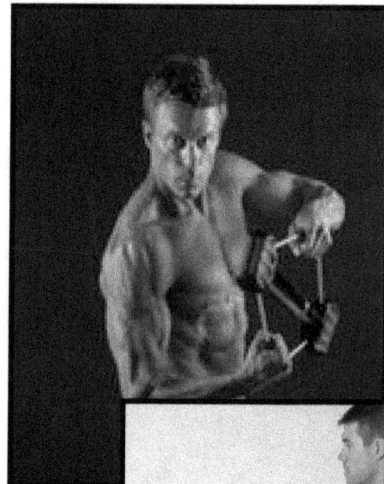

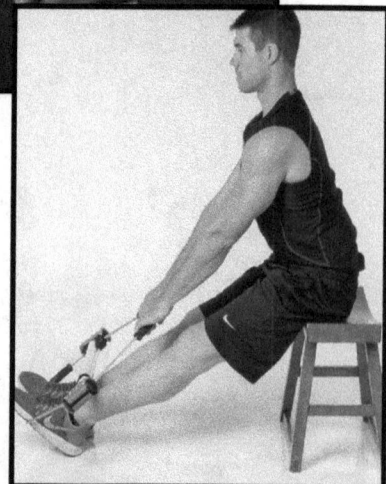

PHASE THREE 30X20

09 REP RANGE POWER PUMP 30 PROGRAM

HOW TO PERFORM THIS ROUTINE:
PHASE TWO 30x20 PHASE

Perform 30 reps followed by a 20 second isometric contraction.
3 sets per exercise

DAY TWO

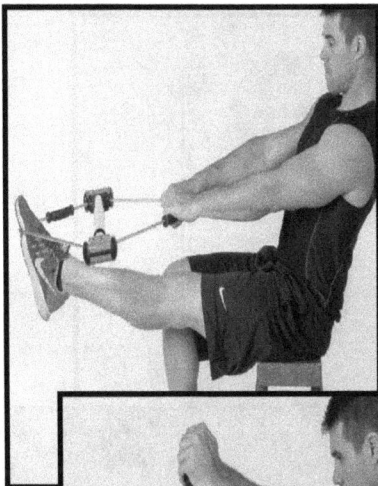

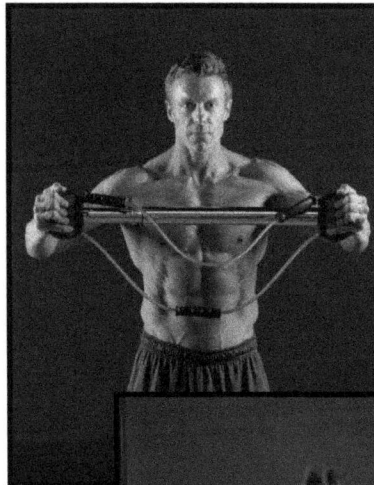

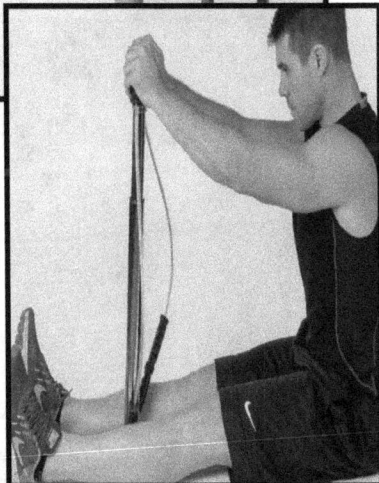

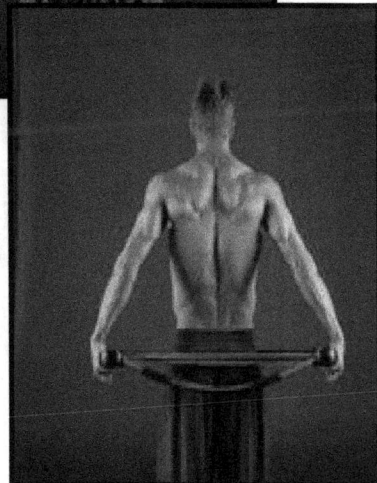

PHASE THREE 30X20

09 REP RANGE POWER PUMP 30 PROGRAM

HOW TO PERFORM THIS ROUTINE:
PHASE TWO 30x20 PHASE

Perform 30 reps followed by a 20 second isometric contraction.
3 sets per exercise

DAY TWO continued...........

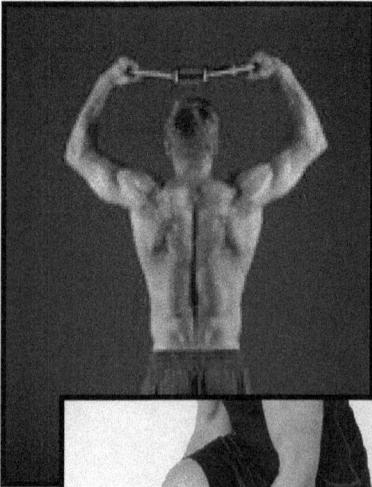

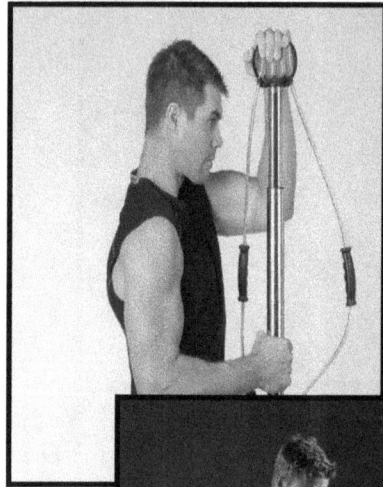

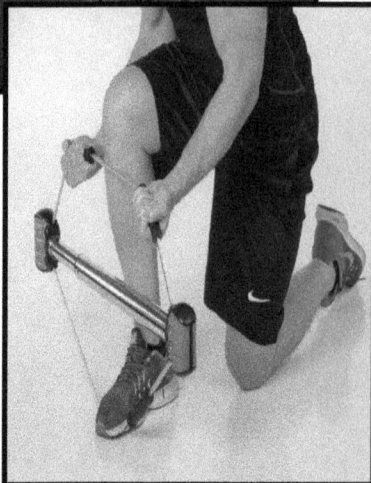

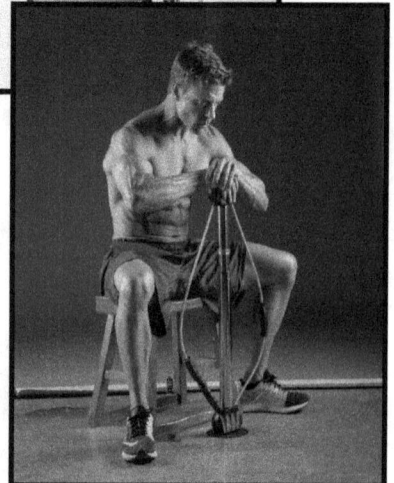

CHAPTER 10
REP RANGE II
MAX-SIZE 40
PHASE 13

PERFORM 40 REPS, HOLD LAST REP 10 SECONDS

MAX SIZE 40 PROGRAM

10 MAX SIZE 40 PROGRAM

HOW TO PERFORM THIS ROUTINE:
MAX SIZE 40 PROGRAM

Perform the **MAX SIZE 40 WORKOUT**—by performing 40 reps. Final rep is held for 10 seconds. Perform all exercises one after the other until all exercises are completed without rest. Perform 3 rounds of these. Rest for 5 seconds before starting the round again.
Alternate day one and day two for 6 days per week.

DAY ONE

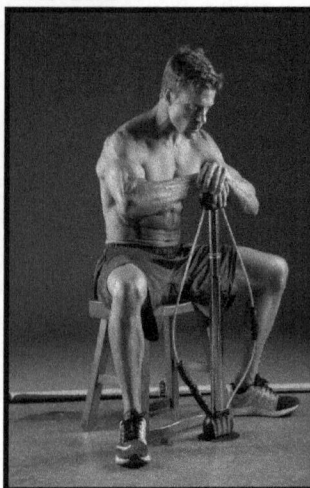
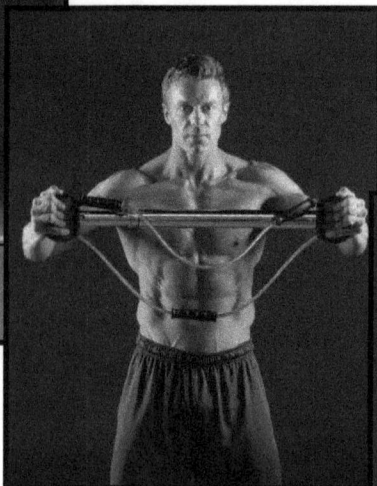
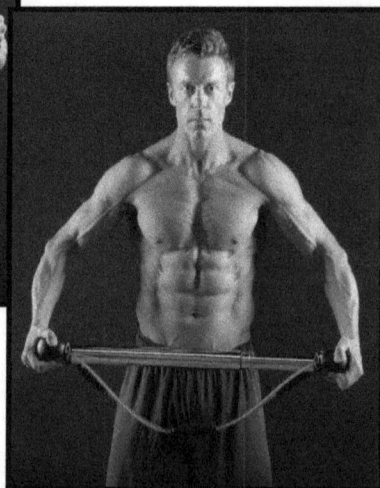

MAX SIZE 40 PROGRAM

10 MAX SIZE 40 PROGRAM

HOW TO PERFORM THIS ROUTINE:
MAX SIZE 40 PROGRAM

Perform the **MAX SIZE 40 WORKOUT**—by performing 40 reps. Final rep is held for 10 seconds. Perform all exercises one after the other until all exercises are completed without rest. Perform 3 rounds of these. Rest for 5 seconds before starting the round again.
Alternate day one and day two for 6 days per week.

DAY ONE continued..........

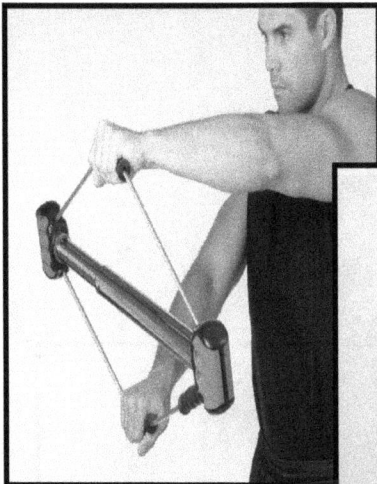

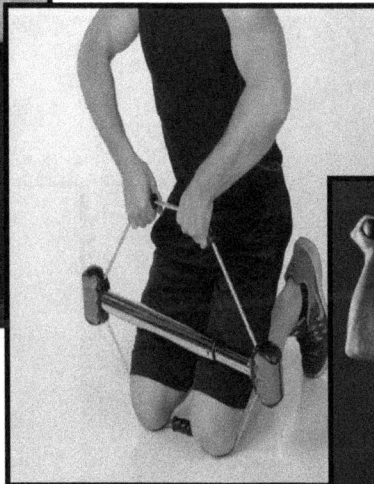

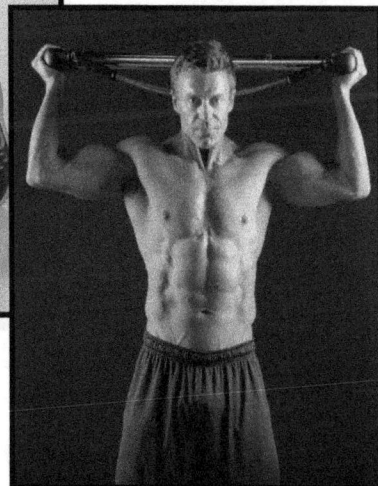

MAX SIZE 40 PROGRAM

10 MAX SIZE 40 PROGRAM

HOW TO PERFORM THIS ROUTINE:
MAX SIZE 40 PROGRAM

Perform the **MAX SIZE 40 WORKOUT**—by performing 40 reps. Final rep is held for 10 seconds. Perform all exercises one after the other until all exercises are completed without rest. Perform 3 rounds of these. Rest for 5 seconds before starting the round again.
Alternate day one and day two for 6 days per week.

DAY ONE continued......

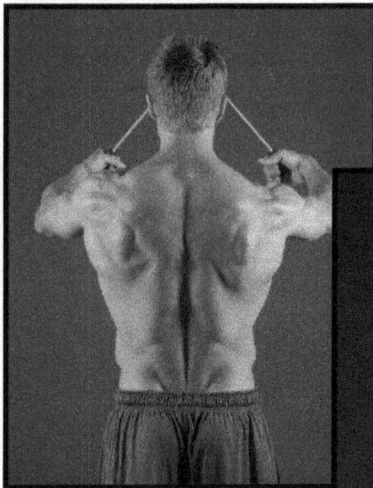

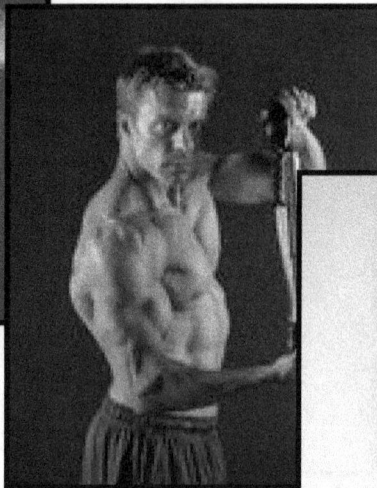

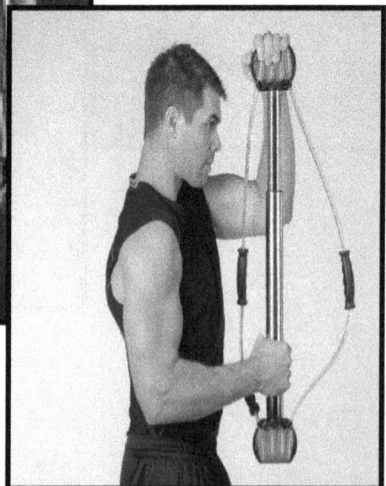

MAX SIZE 40 PROGRAM

10 MAX SIZE 40 PROGRAM

HOW TO PERFORM THIS ROUTINE:
MAX SIZE 40 PROGRAM

Perform the **MAX SIZE 40 WORKOUT**—by performing 40 reps. Final rep is held for 10 seconds. Perform all exercises one after the other until all exercises are completed without rest. Perform 3 rounds of these. Rest for 5 seconds before starting the round again.
Alternate day one and day two for 6 days per week.

DAY TWO

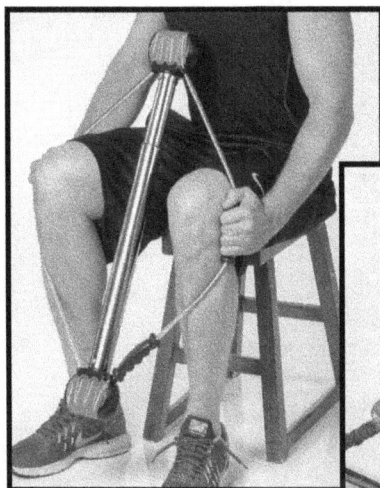
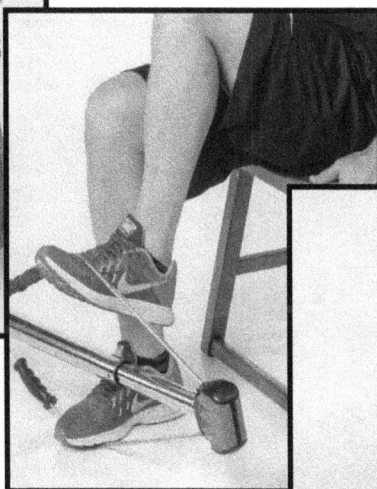
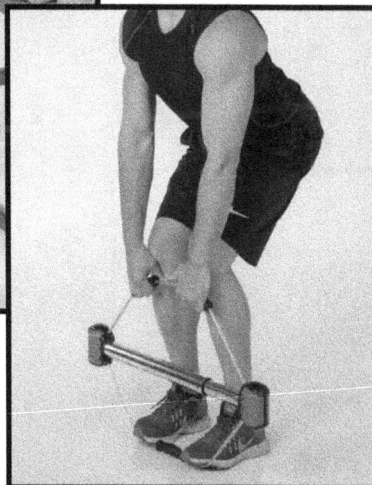

MAX SIZE 40 PROGRAM

10 MAX SIZE 40 PROGRAM

HOW TO PERFORM THIS ROUTINE:
MAX SIZE 40 PROGRAM

Perform the **MAX SIZE 40 WORKOUT**—by performing 40 reps. Final rep is held for 10 seconds. Perform all exercises one after the other until all exercises are completed without rest. Perform 3 rounds of these. Rest for 5 seconds before starting the round again.
Alternate day one and day two for 6 days per week.

DAY TWO continue........

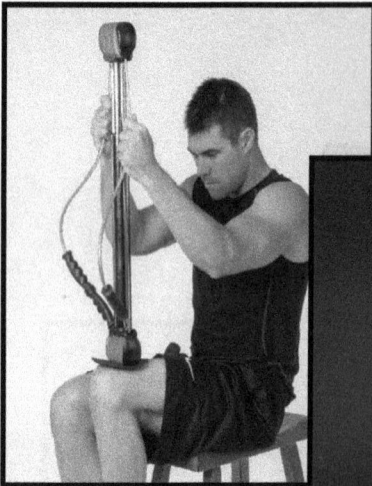

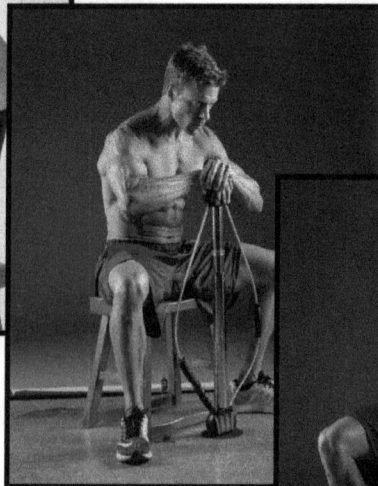

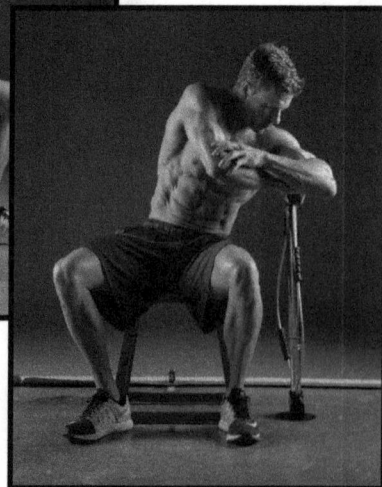

MAX SIZE 40 PROGRAM

10 MAX SIZE 40 PROGRAM

HOW TO PERFORM THIS ROUTINE:
MAX SIZE 40 PROGRAM

Perform the **MAX SIZE 40 WORKOUT**—by performing 40 reps. Final rep is held for 10 seconds. Perform all exercises one after the other until all exercises are completed without rest. Perform 3 rounds of these. Rest for 5 seconds before starting the round again.
Alternate day one and day two for 6 days per week.

DAY TWO continued..........

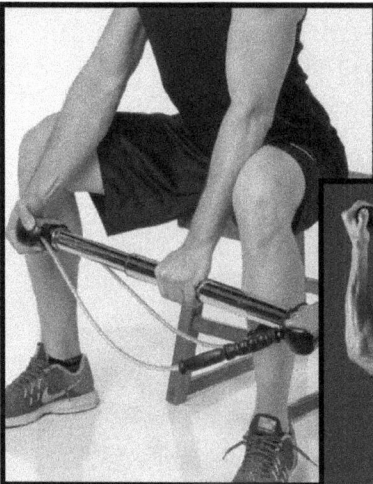

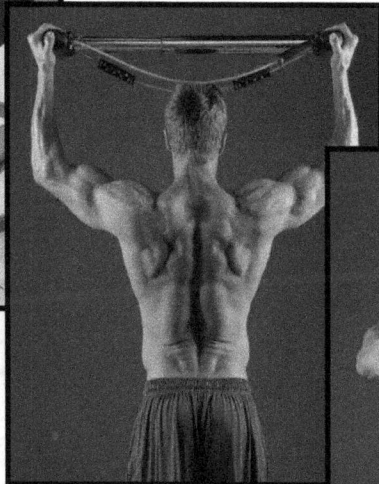

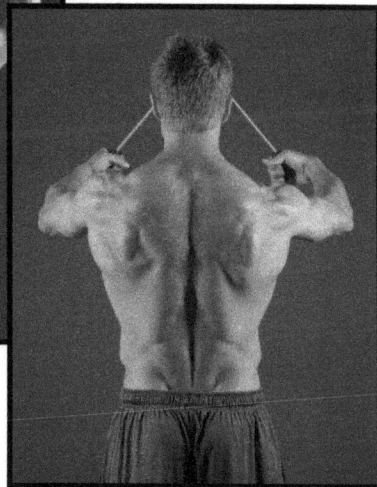

MAX SIZE 40 PROGRAM

10 MAX SIZE 40 PROGRAM

HOW TO PERFORM THIS ROUTINE:
MAX SIZE 40 PROGRAM

Perform the **MAX SIZE 40 WORKOUT**—by performing 40 reps. Final rep is held for 10 seconds. Perform all exercises one after the other until all exercises are completed without rest. Perform 3 rounds of these. Rest for 5 seconds before starting the round again.
Alternate day one and day two for 6 days per week.

DAY TWO continued..........

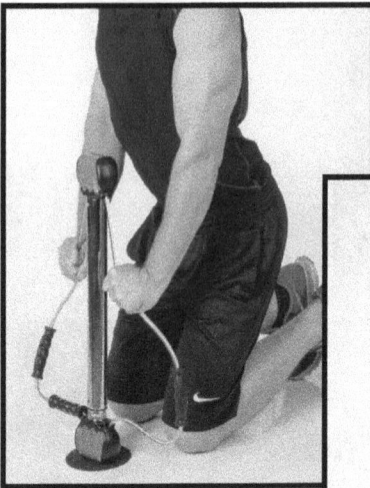

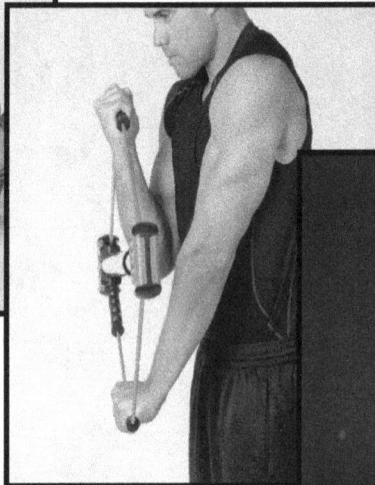

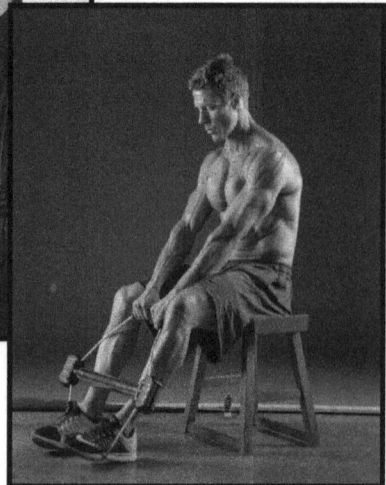

CHAPTER 11
POWER REP WEEK
MAX-HYPER GROWTH
PHASE ONE

REP RANGES CHANGE THROUGHOUT THE WEEK

MAX-HYPER GROWTH PROGRAM

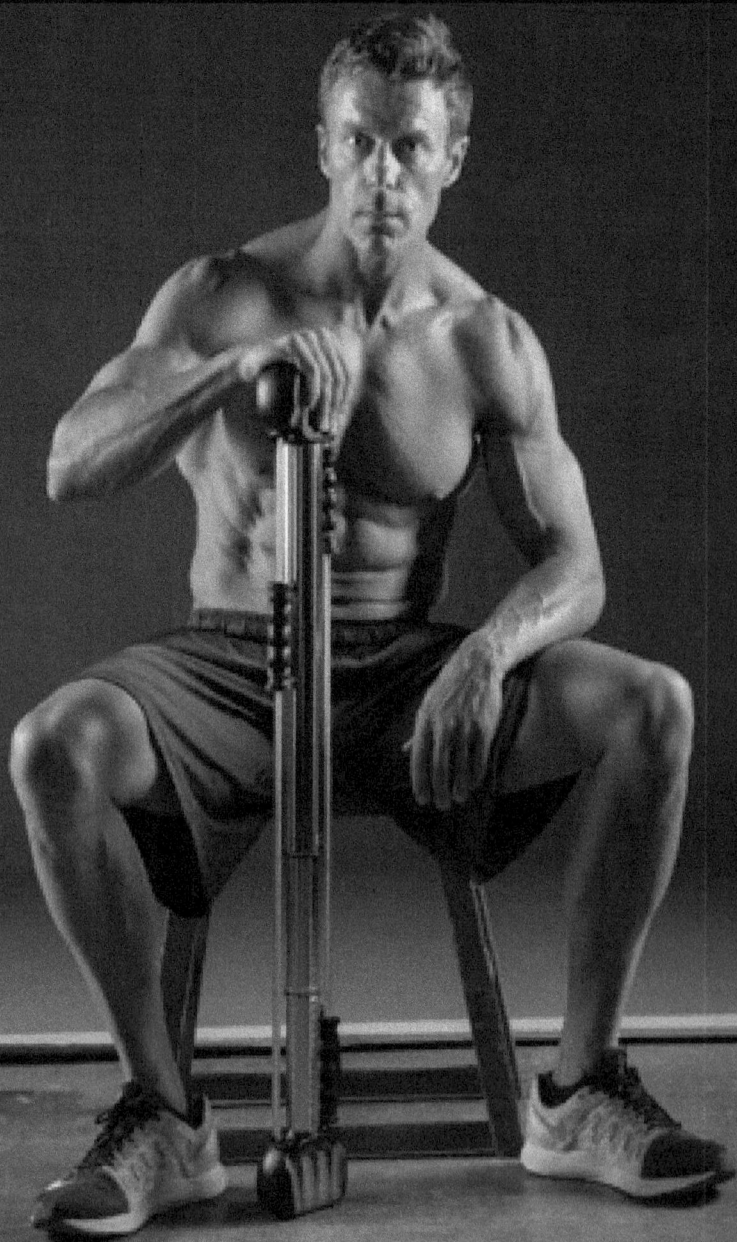

PHASE ONE

11 MAX-HYPER GROWTH PHASE ONE

HOW TO PERFORM THIS ROUTINE:
MAX-HYPER GROWTH PROGRAM

Day 1=30 reps, Day 2=7-9 reps, Day 3=30 reps, Day 4=30 reps, Day 5=7 reps
Day 6=20 reps, Day 7=30 reps. On the last rep perform a 25 second
Isometric contraction. Perform all exercises without rest for 2 rounds.
Perform this routine every day 7 days per week for 3 weeks

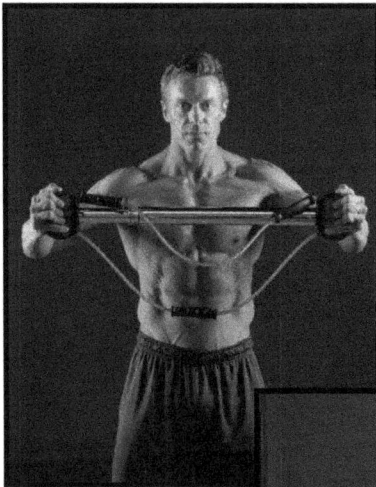

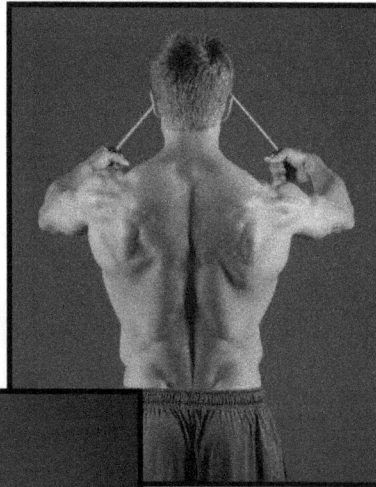

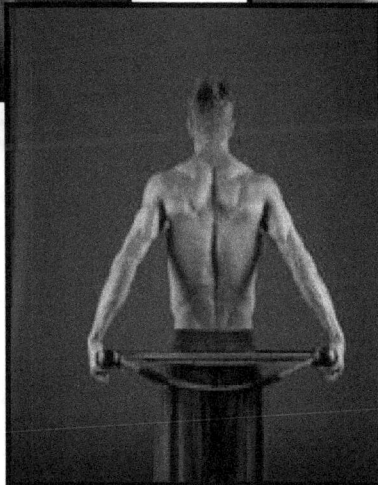

MAX-HYPER GROWTH PROGRAM

11 MAX-HYPER GROWTH PHASE ONE

HOW TO PERFORM THIS ROUTINE:
MAX-HYPER GROWTH PROGRAM

Day 1=30 reps, Day 2=7-9 reps, Day 3=30 reps, Day 4=30 reps, Day 5=7 reps Day 6=20 reps, Day 7=30 reps. On the last rep perform a 25 second Isometric contraction. Perform all exercises without rest for 2 rounds.
Perform this routine every day 7 days per week for 3 weeks

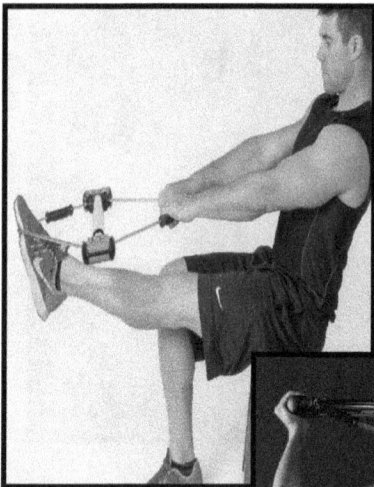

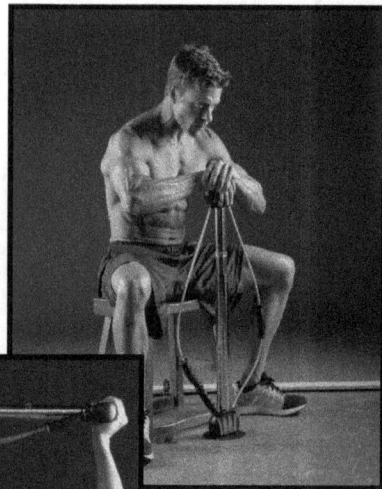

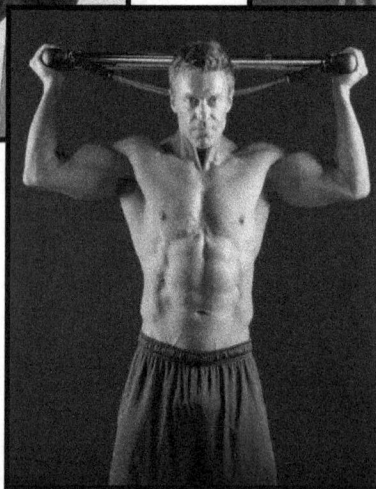

MAX-HYPER GROWTH PROGRAM

11 MAX-HYPER GROWTH PHASE ONE

HOW TO PERFORM THIS ROUTINE:
MAX-HYPER GROWTH PROGRAM

Day 1=30 reps, Day 2=7-9 reps, Day 3=30 reps, Day 4=30 reps, Day 5=7 reps Day 6=20 reps, Day 7=30 reps. On the last rep perform a 25 second Isometric contraction. Perform all exercises without rest for 2 rounds.
Perform this routine every day 7 days per week for 3 weeks

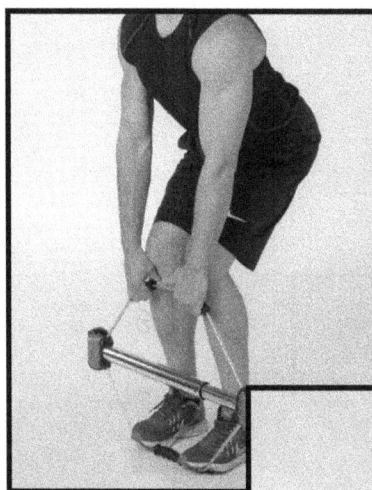

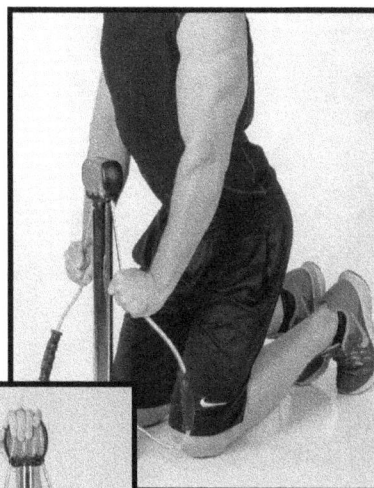

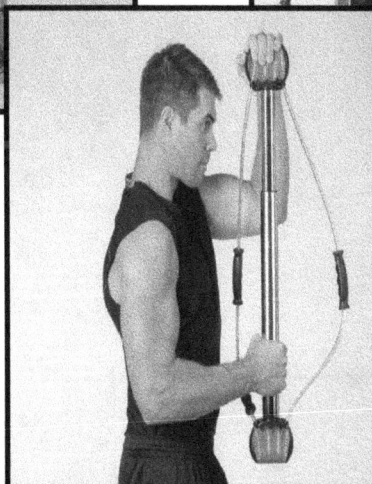

PHASE TWO

11 MAX-HYPER GROWTH PHASE TWO

HOW TO PERFORM THIS ROUTINE:
MAX-HYER GROWTH PROGRAM

Day 1=12reps, Day 2=10 reps, Day 3=40 reps, Day 4=40 reps, Day 5=7 reps
Day 6=5 reps, Day 7=40 reps. On the last rep perform a 20 second
Isometric contraction. Perform all exercises without rest for 2 rounds.
Perform this routine every day 7 days per week for 3 weeks

DAY ONE

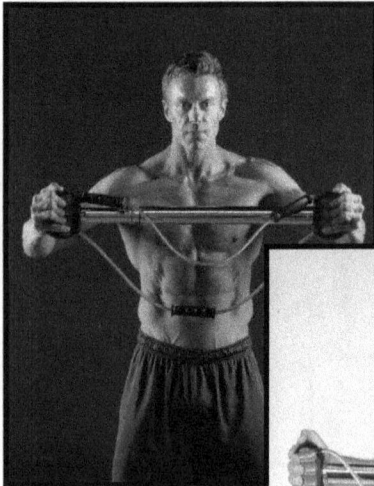
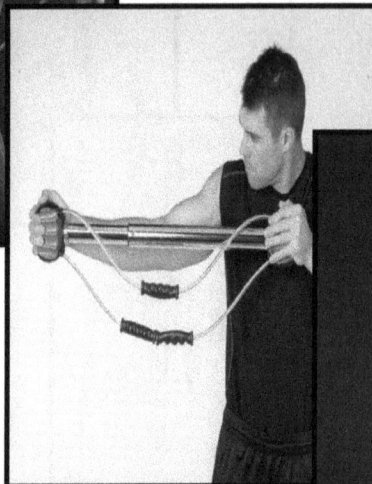
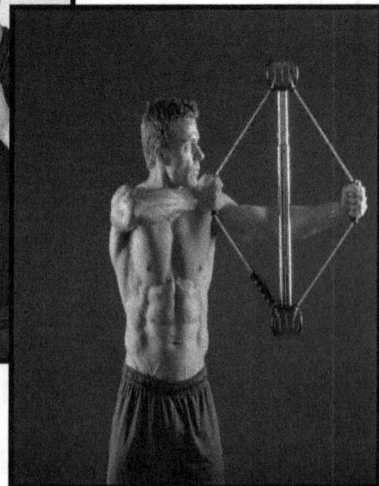

PHASE TWO

11 MAX-HYPER GROWTH PHASE TWO

HOW TO PERFORM THIS ROUTINE:
MAX-HYER GROWTH PROGRAM

Day 1=12 reps, Day 2=10 reps, Day 3=40 reps, Day 4=40 reps, Day 5=7 reps
Day 6=5 reps, Day 7=40 reps. On the last rep perform a 20 second
Isometric contraction. Perform all exercises without rest for 2 rounds.
Perform this routine every day 7 days per week for 3 weeks

DAY ONE continued..........

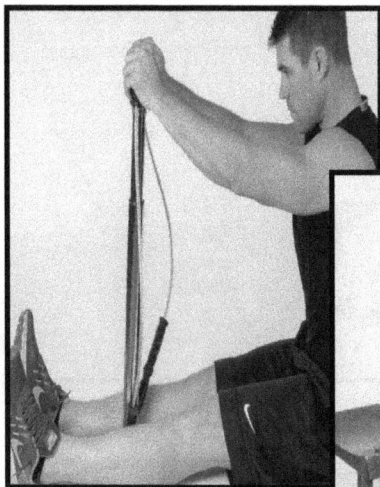

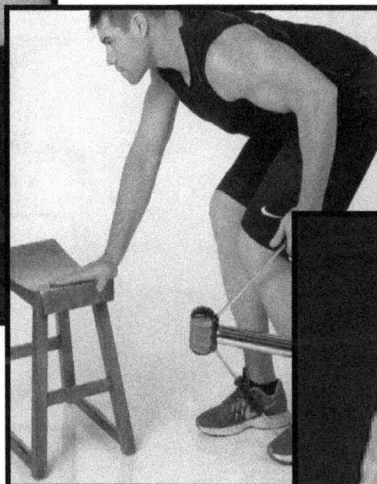

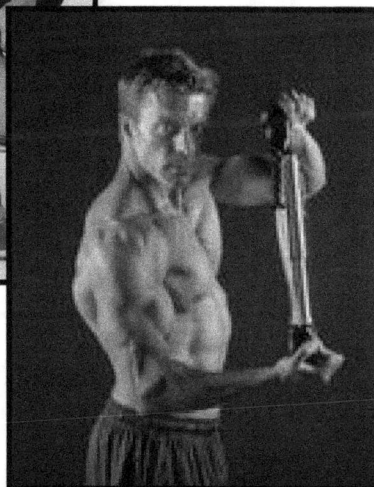

PHASE TWO

11 MAX-HYPER GROWTH PHASE TWO

HOW TO PERFORM THIS ROUTINE:
MAX-HYER GROWTH PROGRAM

Day 1=12reps, Day 2=10 reps, Day 3=40 reps, Day 4=40 reps, Day 5=7 reps
Day 6=5 reps, Day 7=40 reps. On the last rep perform a 20 second
Isometric contraction. Perform all exercises without rest for 2 rounds.
Perform this routine every day 7 days per week for 3 weeks

DAY ONE contin........

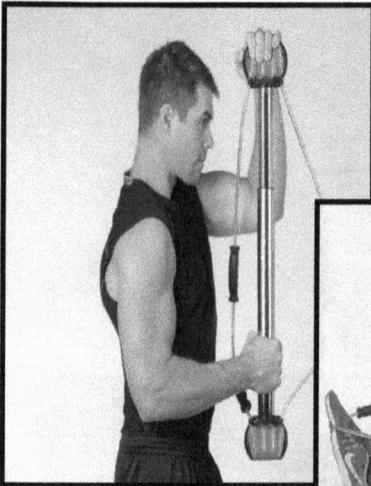

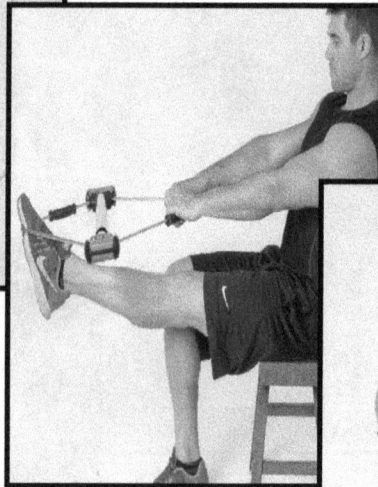

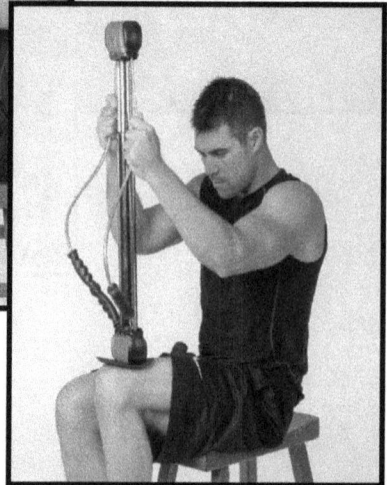

PHASE TWO

11 MAX-HYPER GROWTH PHASE TWO

HOW TO PERFORM THIS ROUTINE:
MAX-HYER GROWTH PROGRAM

Day 1=12reps, Day 2=10 reps, Day 3=40 reps, Day 4=40 reps, Day 5=7 reps
Day 6=5 reps, Day 7=40 reps. On the last rep perform a 20 second
Isometric contraction. Perform all exercises without rest for 2 rounds.
Perform this routine every day 7 days per week for 3 weeks

DAY TWO

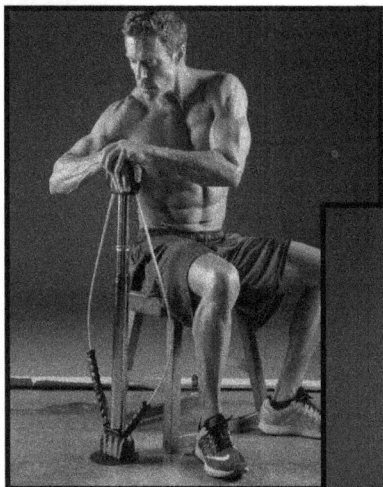
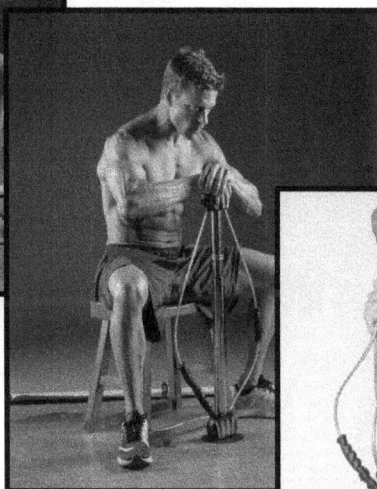
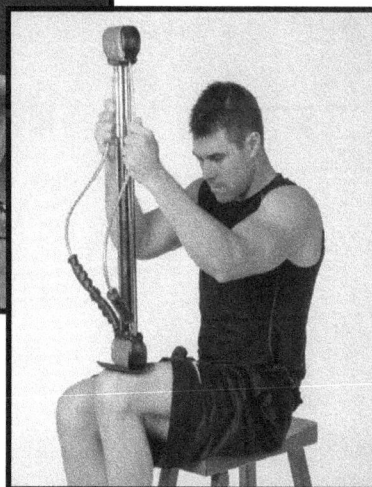

PHASE TWO

11 MAX-HYPER GROWTH PHASE TWO

HOW TO PERFORM THIS ROUTINE:
MAX-HYER GROWTH PROGRAM

Day 1=12reps, Day 2=10 reps, Day 3=40 reps, Day 4=40 reps, Day 5=7 reps
Day 6=5 reps, Day 7=40 reps. On the last rep perform a 20 second
Isometric contraction. Perform all exercises without rest for 2 rounds.
Perform this routine every day 7 days per week for 3 weeks

DAY TWO continued...........

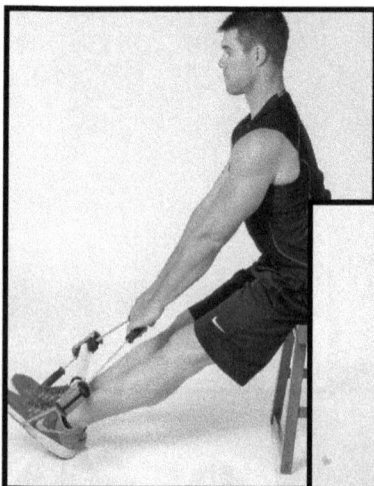

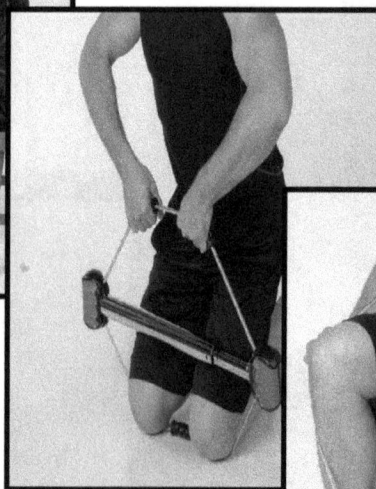

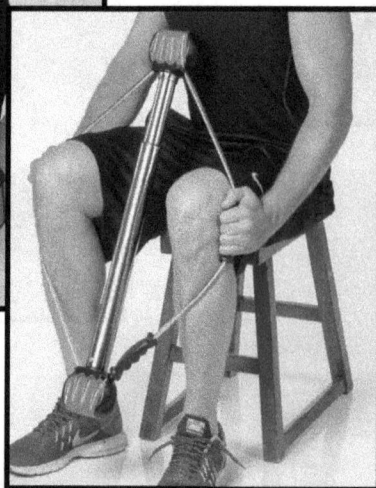

PHASE TWO

11 MAX-HYPER GROWTH PHASE TWO

HOW TO PERFORM THIS ROUTINE:
MAX-HYER GROWTH PROGRAM

Day 1=12reps, Day 2=10 reps, Day 3=40 reps, Day 4=40 reps, Day 5=7 reps
Day 6=5 reps, Day 7=40 reps. On the last rep perform a 20 second
Isometric contraction. Perform all exercises without rest for 2 rounds.
Perform this routine every day 7 days per week for 3 weeks

DAY TWO continued...........

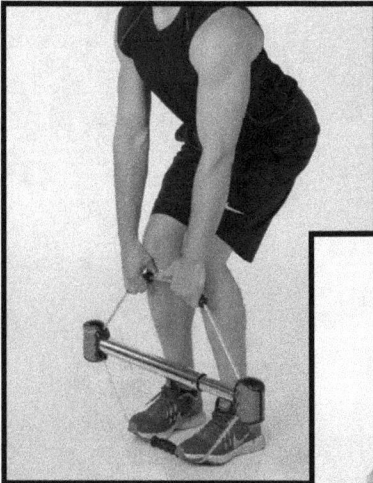

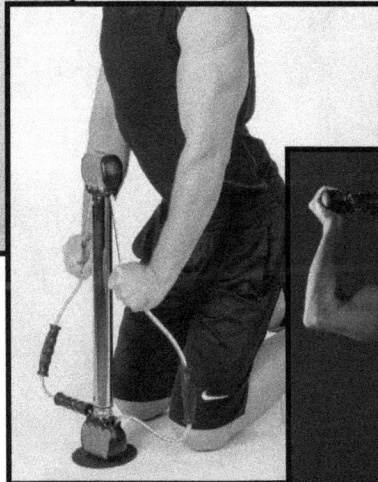

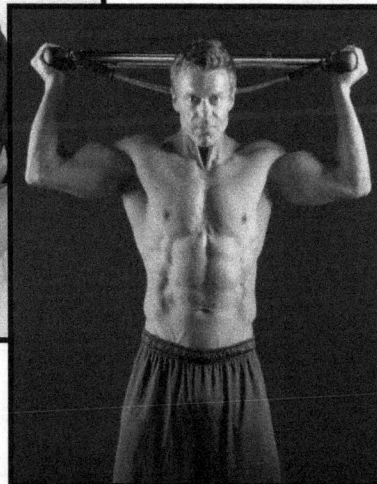

Looking forward to hearing from you on your progress. Please drop me an email skippymarl@icloud.com

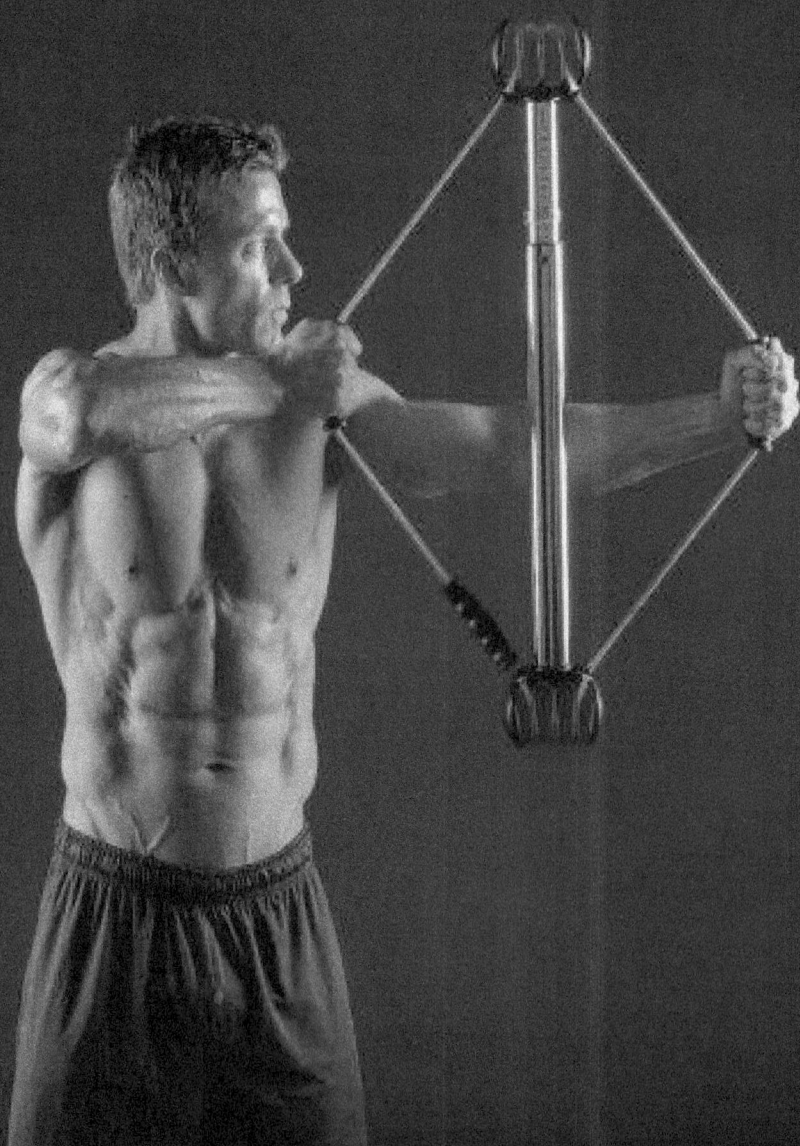

MOST IMPROVED STUDENT AWARD
COMING SOON
JUNE 25th 2020